80 Cool Haircuts for the Latest Thin Hair

Everyone desires to have rich hair that is obedient in style and constantly looks excellent. However, the secret to a genuinely easy trendy appearance is in the appropriate haircut. Even with inadequate hair thickness and density, you may come up with some incredibly gorgeous designs.

Step into the world of amazing hairstyles by reading through the handpicked gallery of photographs displaying the greatest haircuts for thin hair. You are guaranteed to uncover a selection of inventive methods and style hacks to add volume and texture to thin locks.

GRACE E. KHOURY

Introduction

there's no need to stick especially to shorter durations. Good hair stylists have strategies on how to make your thin hair look thicker even in lengthy haircuts.

Whether you desire lengthy strands that you can sling over your shoulder or a fast and simple short style, we have 80 haircuts for thin hair that will suit your preferences. Thin hair might seem lifeless and uninspired if it is not done appropriately. Pump up the volume on uninteresting hair with a textured bob, glossy layers or full curls!

Table of Contents

GRACE E. KHOURY

Perfect Short Haircut for Fine Hair

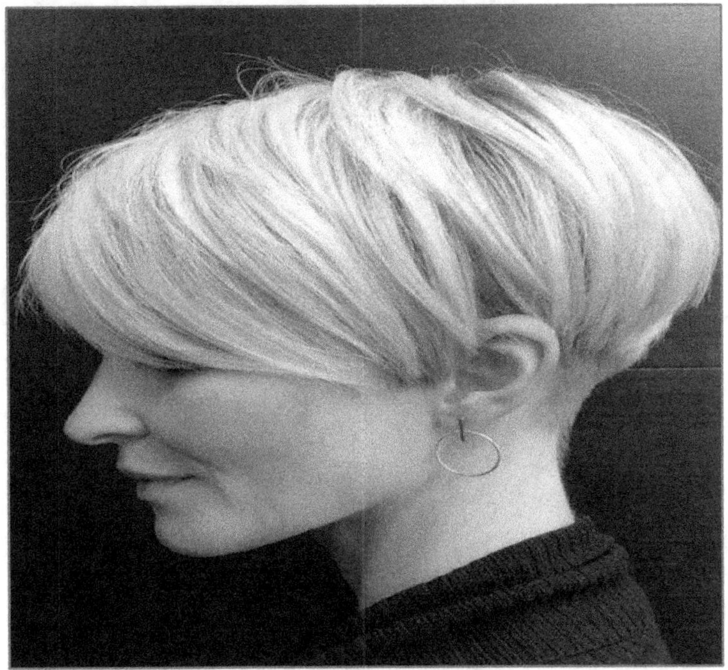

A perfect illusion of a beautiful short haircut can be achieved by adding extra volume to the top and trimming the sides and back. The blondish highlights give the side-swept hair dimension and emphasize its rough texture—a fantastic neatly carefree style! As you can see, layering, highlights, choppy ends, and a destructured appearance all work well for volume at any length. I hope that gives you some great ideas!

GRACE E. KHOURY 7

Brushed-Over Blunt Bob Haircut

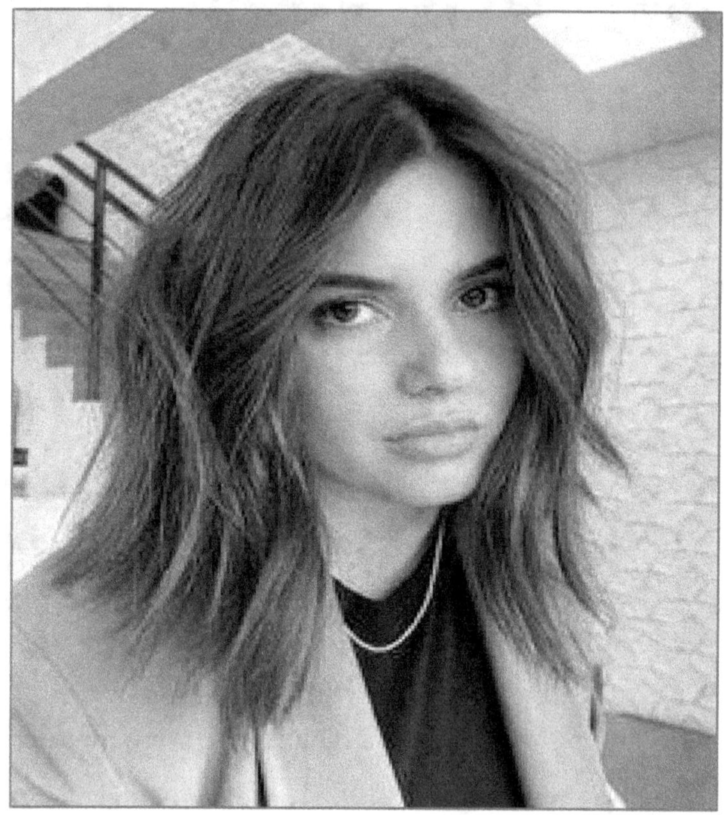

When worn with spectacles, this look epitomizes "casual cool." You only need to flip your hair to leave! Put on a stylish pair of sunglasses for a carefree weekend style.

Messy Long Bob for Thin Hair

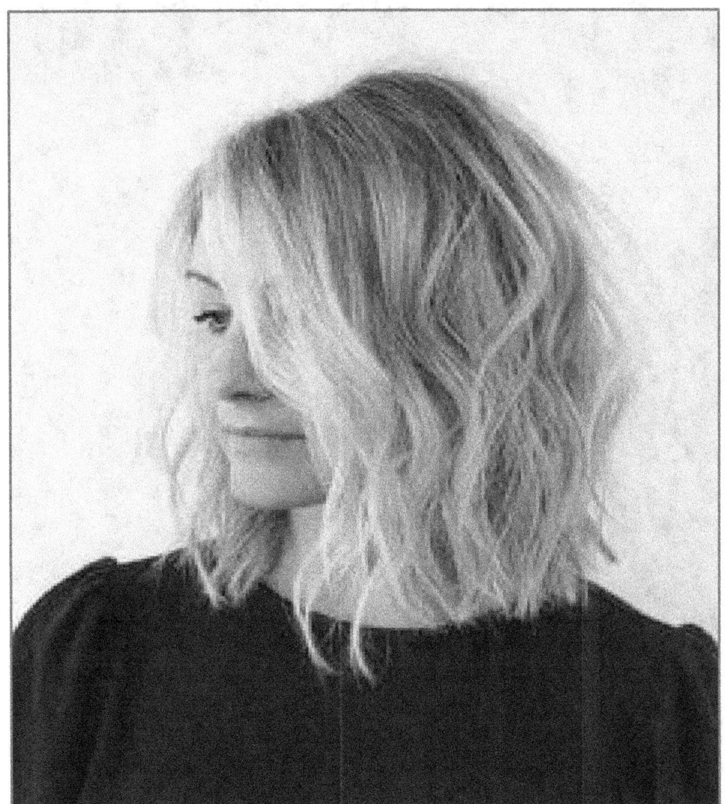

The picture of carefree elegance is a tousled lob. The hair that comes from rolling out of bed doesn't always look like this, though. Use hairspray to set fantastically messy hairstyles for fine hair by teasing the roots!

Arctic White Textured Bob

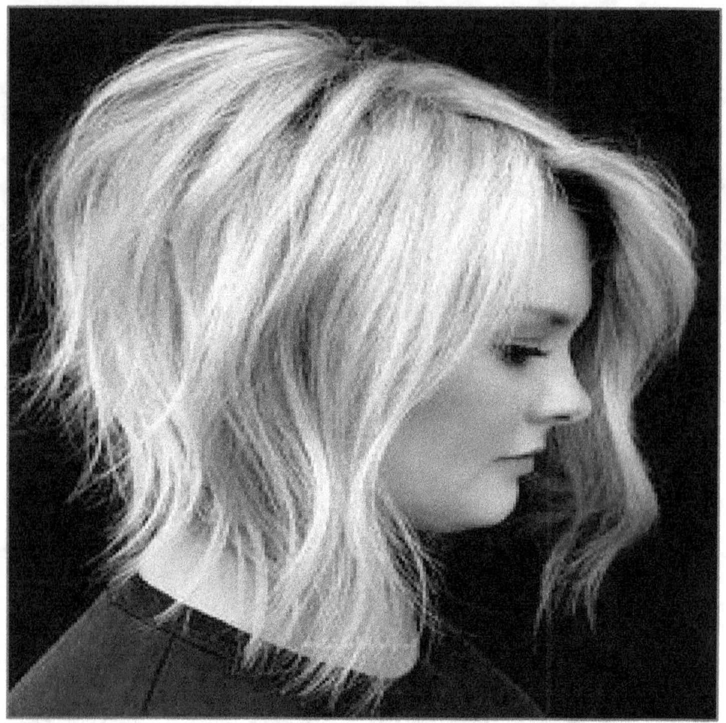

When thinking about bobs for thin hair, colour is crucial. As long as the shoulder-length cut is textured, going arctic white (a solid, flat shade) is possible. Adding grey or silver undertones is a clever strategy that gives fine hair depth.

Messy Bob for Thin Hair

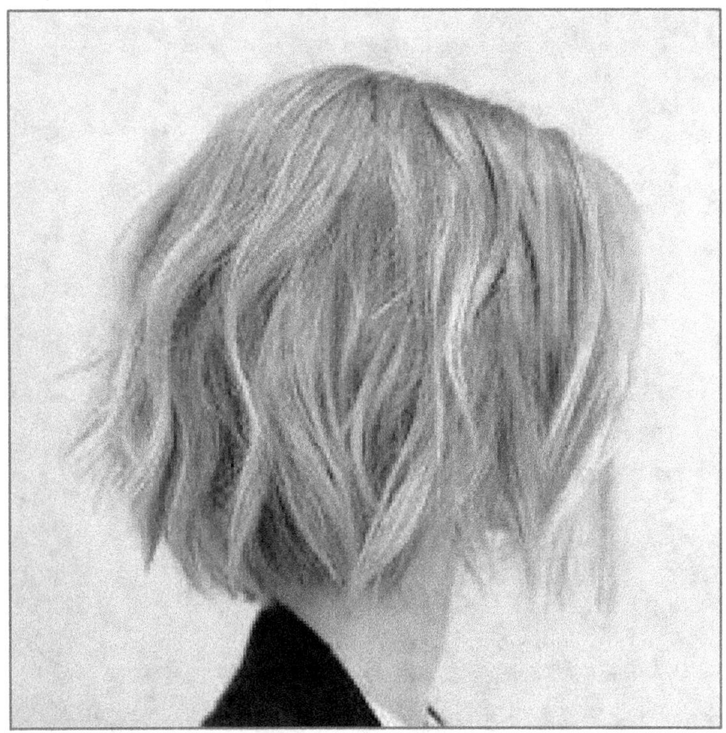

It might be really difficult to have fine hair, but on the plus side, thin hair looks great with messier hairstyles! Put your flat iron away and increase the volume of your texturizing products, particularly ones that are designed to add volume.

Light Layered Cut with Balayage

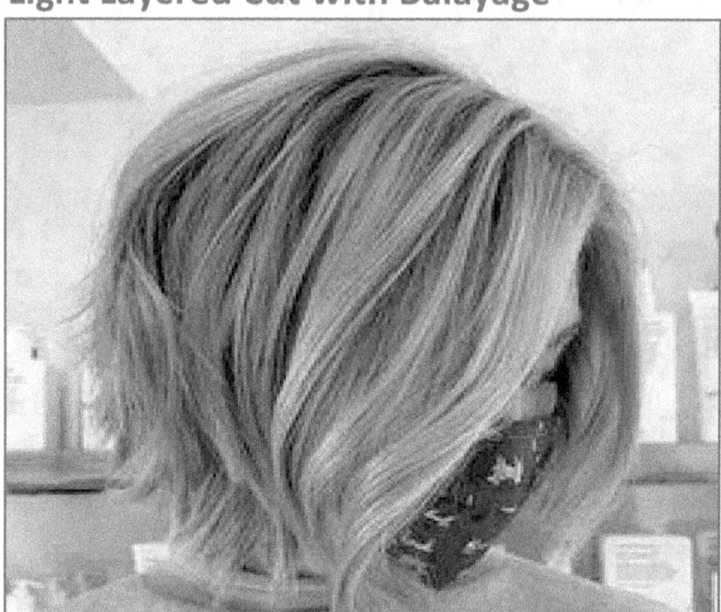

Your hair will bounce and appear larger and more voluminous thanks to layers. Try balayage or ombre with bleached top layers and ends to improve this effect. The lightness and femininity of this look are ethereal, and thin hair can benefit much from the correct colour and cut!

Warm Copper Balayage for Medium Hair

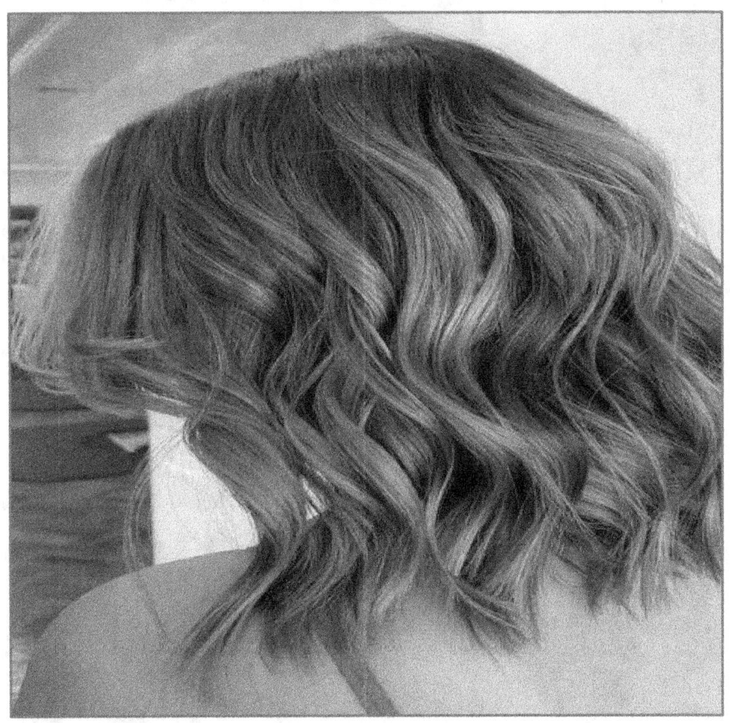

Is there anything more stunning than this balayage of warm copper? A warm tone highlight over your neutral base hair colour will make manes look richer and consequently thicker. Take a walk on the warmer side if you have naturally ashy skin tones to counteract fine hair.

Razored Bob with Waves and Blonde Balayage

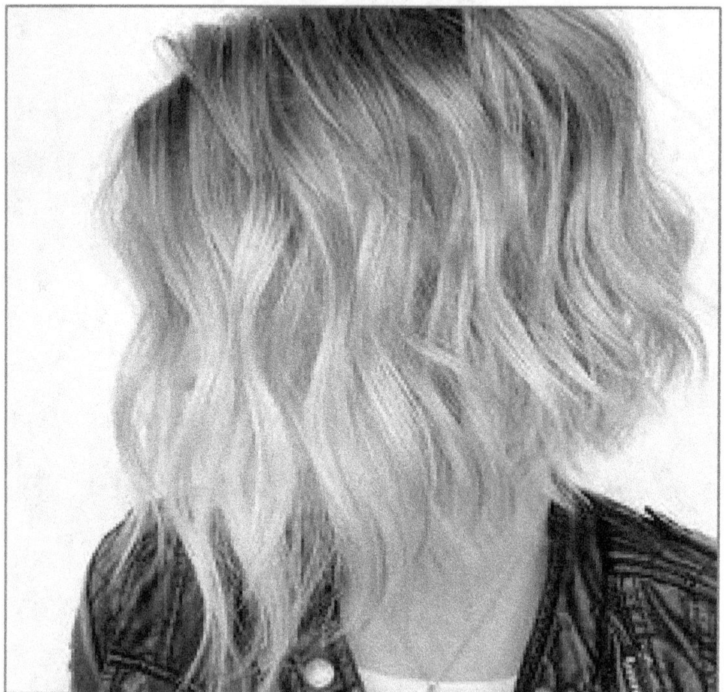

Because they reduce the width of big features, long face-framing pieces are flattering for round face shapes. If the length falls below the chin, they also soften the sharp characteristics of square faces.

Blunt Cut for Fine Hair

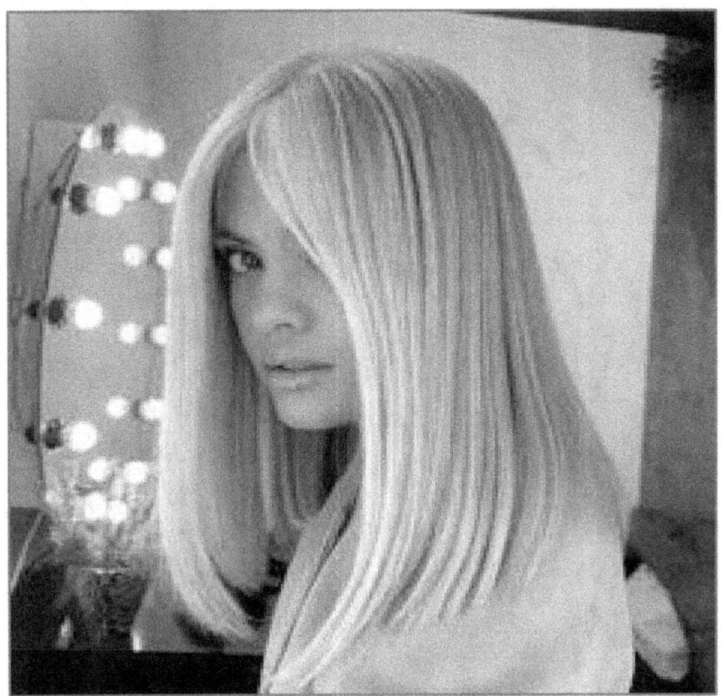

The natural sleekness of fine, straight hair is a major asset. If you want something a little more subdued, volume is not a concern. The simple medium-length cut is certainly elegant and creates an impact even without layers or waves.

Layered Haircut for Thin Hair

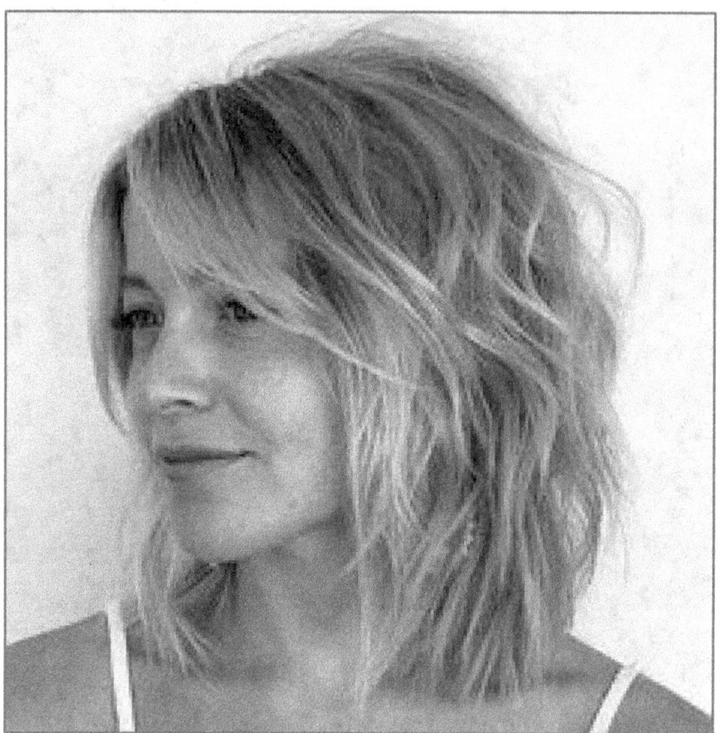

You wouldn't believe it, but medium hairstyles for thin hair may give your mane a large, vibrant look. You'll get the oomph you need with loose, unruly barrel curls paired with layers and side-swept bangs. If you want to seem like a complete bombshell, give this look a try; it is dripping with refinement and sensual style.

Layered Bob with Platinum Balayage

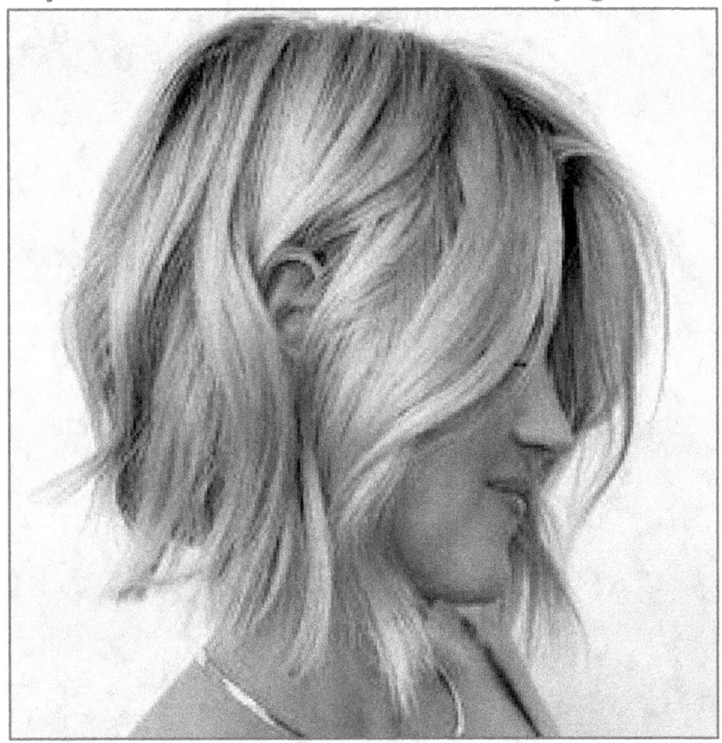

When it comes to clothes, the brighter the bigger they can make you look. While at times you might want to avoid super bright colors, it works as an advantage for fine tresses. It makes them appear fuller and more lustrous. A few layers at the ends will enhance this effect.

Tousled Blunt Brunette Bob

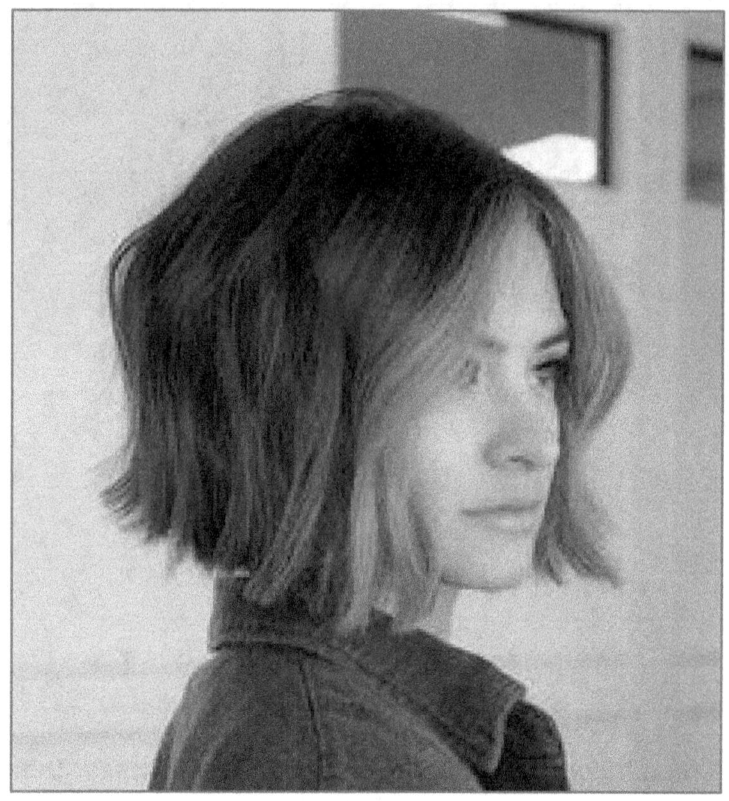

Choose a blunt bob if you're sick of the layered appearance. Give your hair a tousle to avoid the flat appearance that comes with thin hair. Put some hair behind one ear to give it a fuller appearance, and leave a large chunk of hair hanging down in front.

Brown Lob with Piecey Waves and Highlights

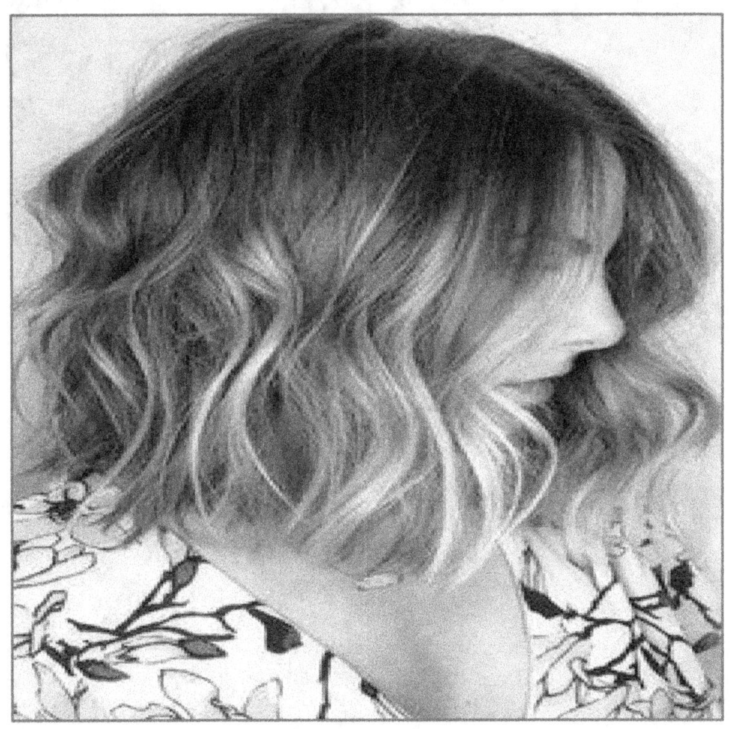

Keep your hair's length, texture, and thickness in mind as you browse hairstyles for thin hair. Given that short hair is naturally lighter than long hair, cropped cuts are better equipped to maintain height and bounce. Graduation down the length may be necessary for longer hair to look more dynamic.

Short Layered Blonde Hairstyle

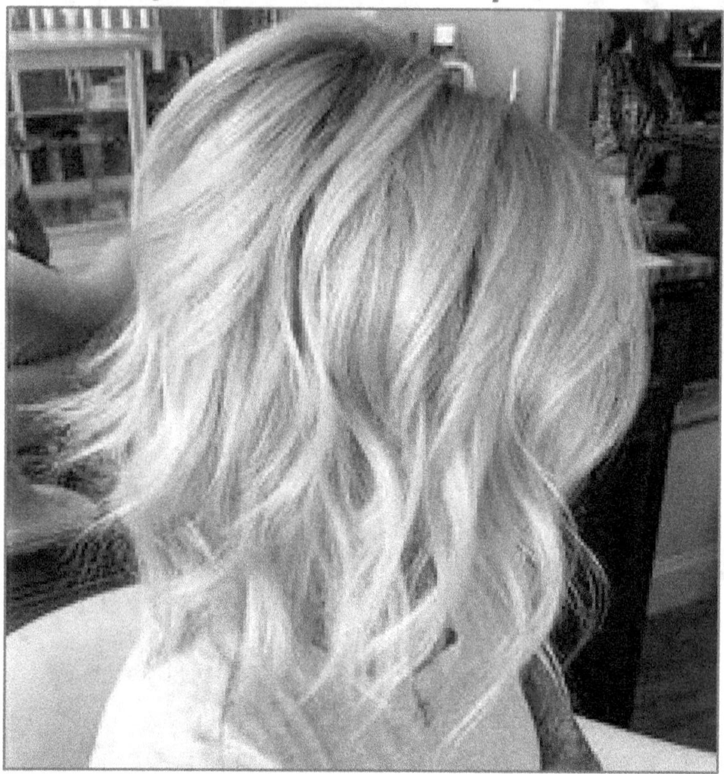

Think about what constitutes your sense of style before selecting one of the bob haircuts for fine hair from what seems like an infinity of alternatives. The short-to-medium length is still chic and professional while the stacked bob is ideal if you want something with a little sass.

Shoulder-Length Wavy Cut with Curtain Bangs

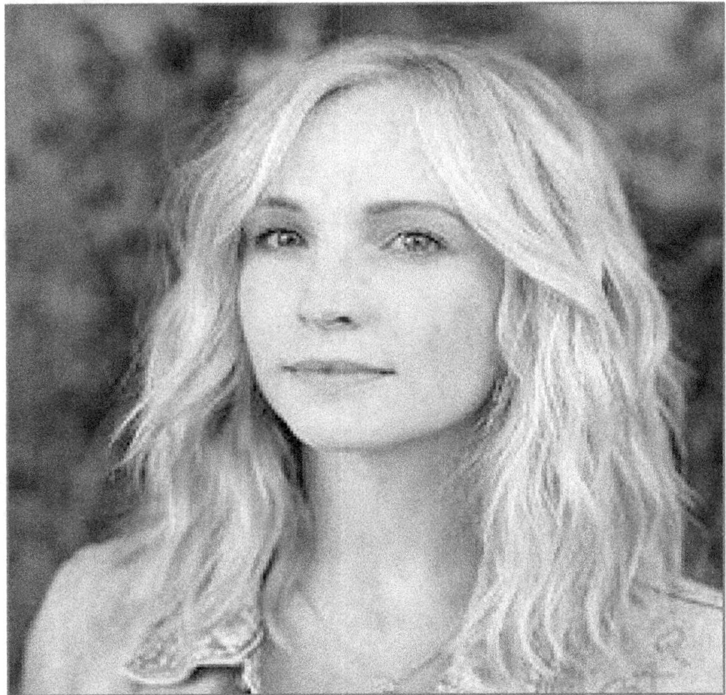

A shoulder-length bob with layers can be styled in a modest updo, curly, wavy, or straight. Finding a high-quality nourishing and restoring hair care solution that is appropriate for your hair type is crucial given all the heat exposure.

Short Bob with Razored Wavy Layers

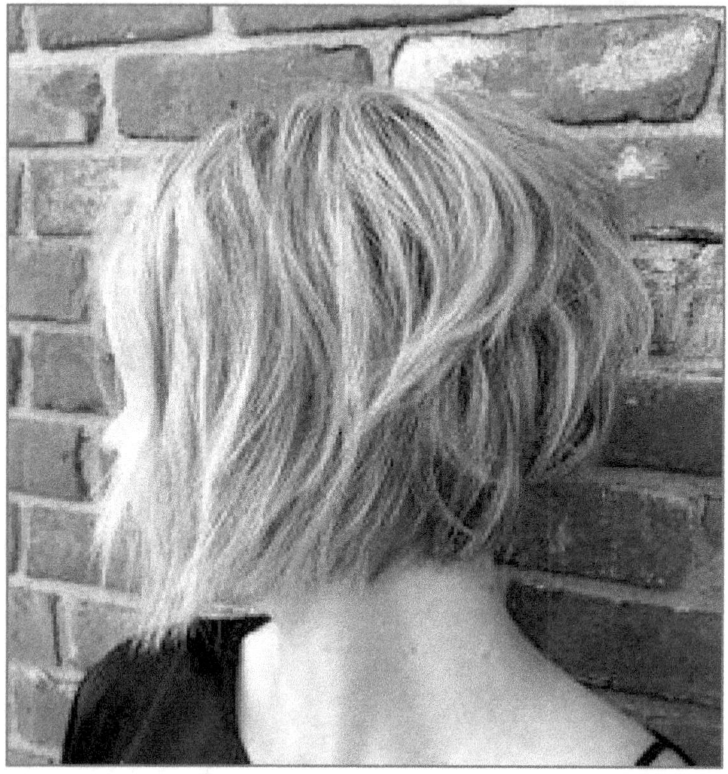

One of the greatest methods is to shave the outer layer of the hair, which highlights the texture and makes the hair blendable without causing hair loss. This haircut makes it easier to manipulate your hair because you can straighten or curl it without having to take heavier, jagged layers into account.

Medium Haircut with Face-Framing Pieces

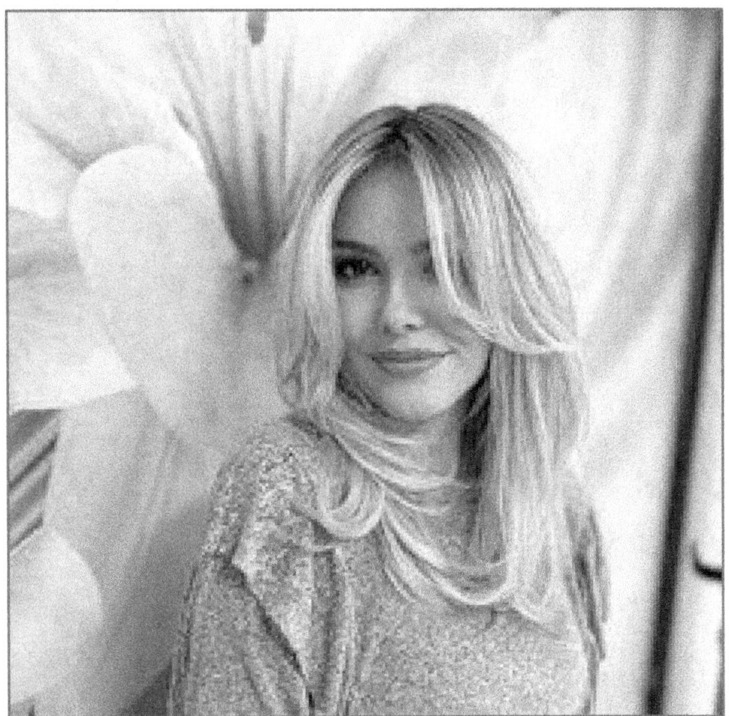

The greatest hairstyles for thin hair are always those with smooth, straight medium-length locks. Below the chin, the face-framing layers cascade down till they reach the shoulders. The rich and elegant colour of the beige-blonde balayage looks lovely and natural on most skin tones.

Disconnected Shaggy Bob with Highlighted Ends

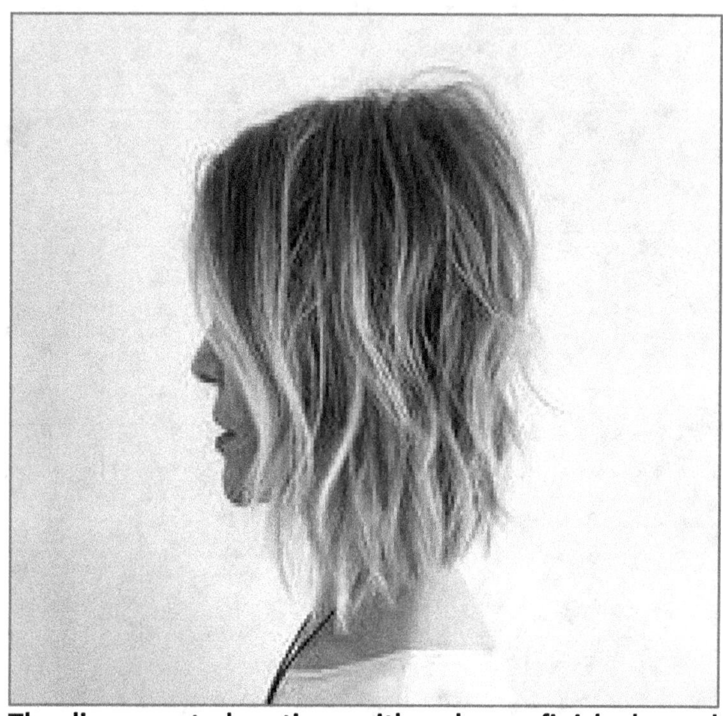

The disconnected sections with a shaggy finish channel a punky vibe. This short layered style is perfectly dressed up by Ombre to spotlight the piecez-ness of the haircut.

Sleek Sharp Bob with an Off-Centered Part

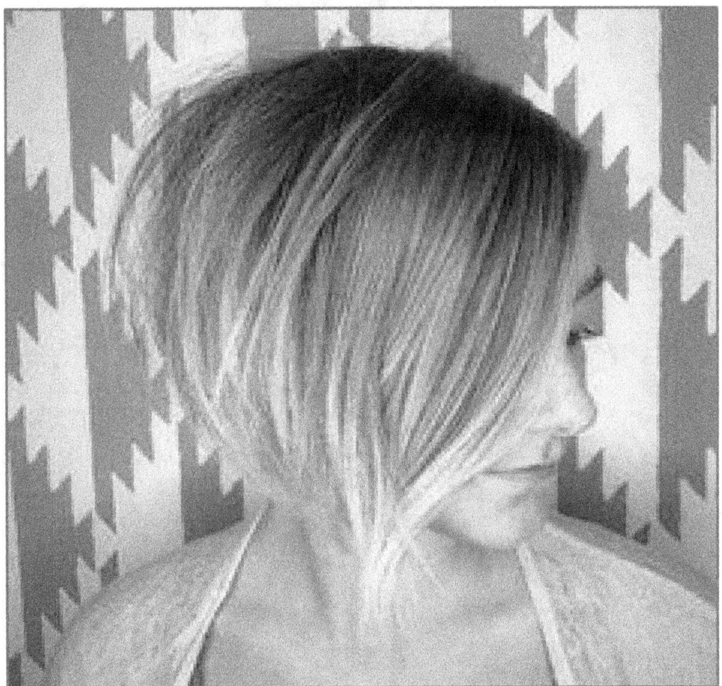

For a sleek and polished chin-length appearance, flat iron thin hair straight rather than trying to volumize it with tight curls. For women with wider cheeks, the locks descending toward the oval face have a slimming effect, and the razored ends add a little bit of substance.

Long Blonde Shag

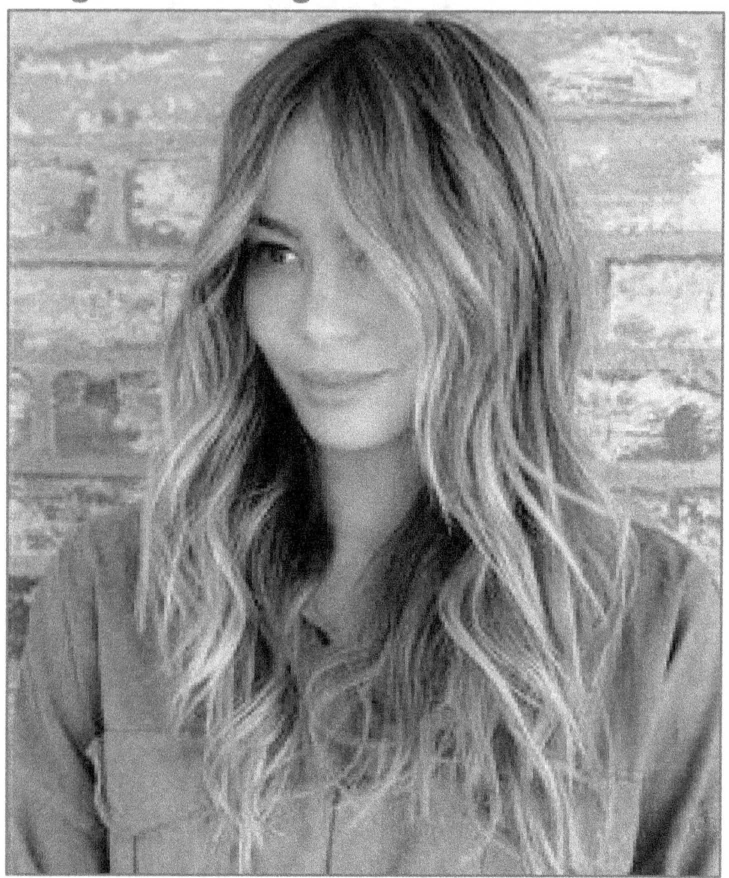

Long hair with lots of waves will help frame your face and give it a somewhat rounder appearance if it is angular and thin. When parted in the middle and little messy, this long, blonde shag looks fantastic.

Shoulder Length Haircut with Deep Side Bang

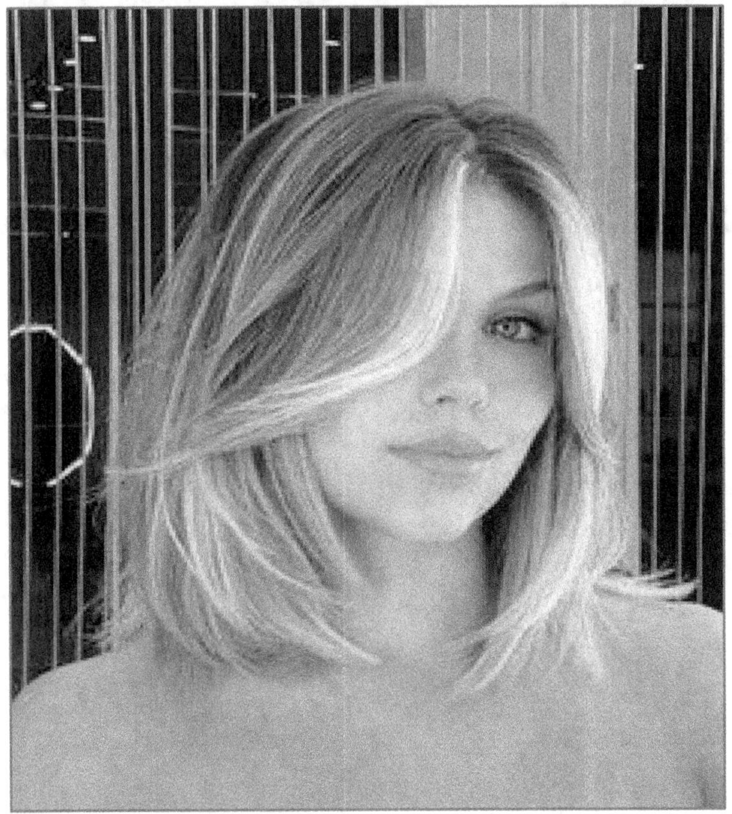

The deep side part adds intrigue and prevents the style from looking flat and dull while the shoulder length cut with light layers adds some sass to the lovely blonde shade.

Shattered Bronde Pixie Bob

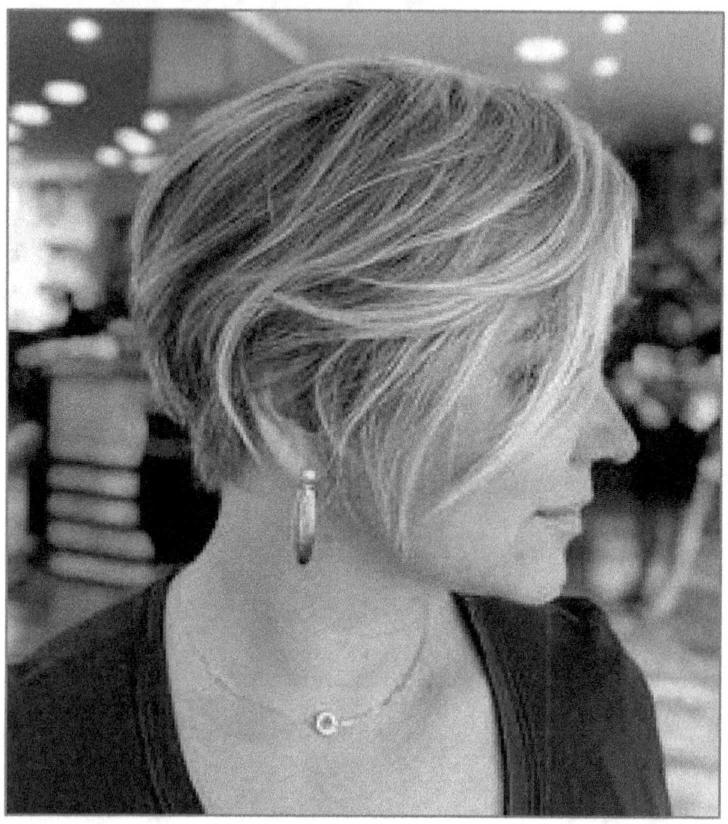

An overgrown pixie is a popular style for women who have very thin hair. Let your locks grow out to the desired length, and then chop the ends. For an extra sexy vibe, part your hair on the side and comb the extra-long, chin-length bangs to fall in front of one eye.

Mid-Length Wavy Cut with Wispy Layers

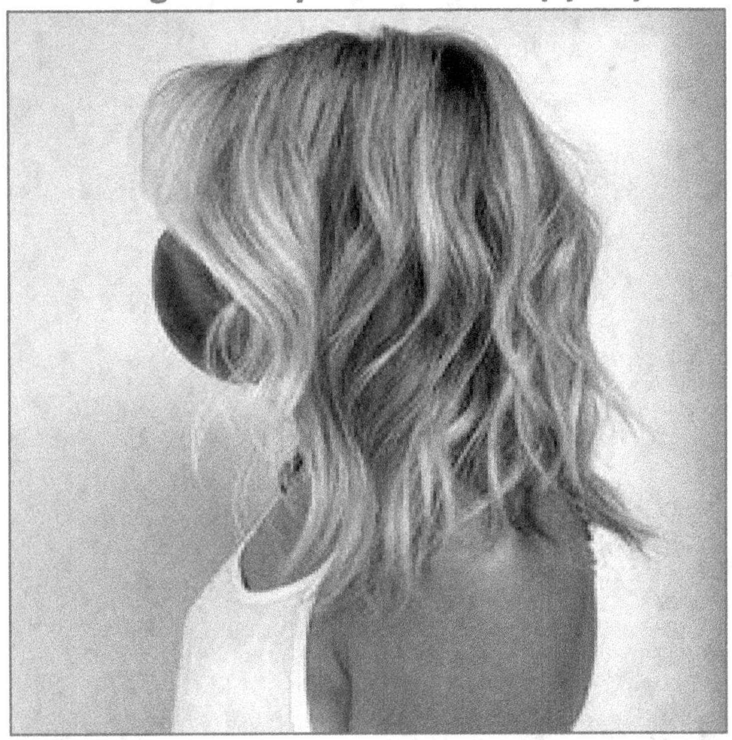

If your short bob has successfully grown out, you're probably ready for one of these adorable mid-length hairstyles for thin-haired women. It's a delicate, layered style that brings out the best in your waves and looks beautiful parted either on the side or down the center. The modest form is given vitality by the color of sun-kissed golden blonde.

Textured Haircut for Short Hair

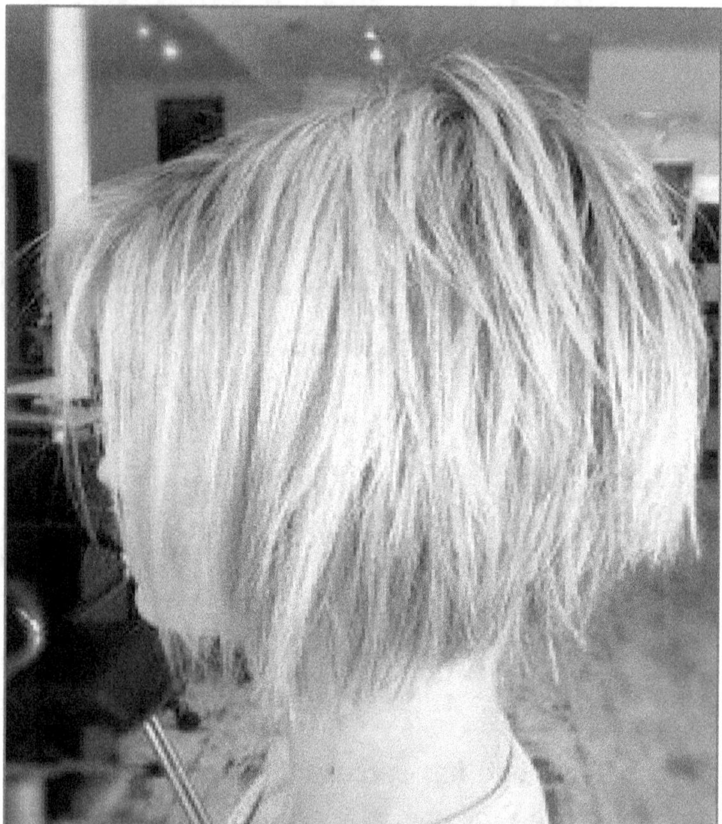

Chopping off dead ends is one of the finest ways to encourage thinning hair to grow. Frequent breaks have a cascading impact and can prevent healthy components from thriving. Cut the hair at an angle to hasten growth!

Bronzed Blonde Bob Blowout

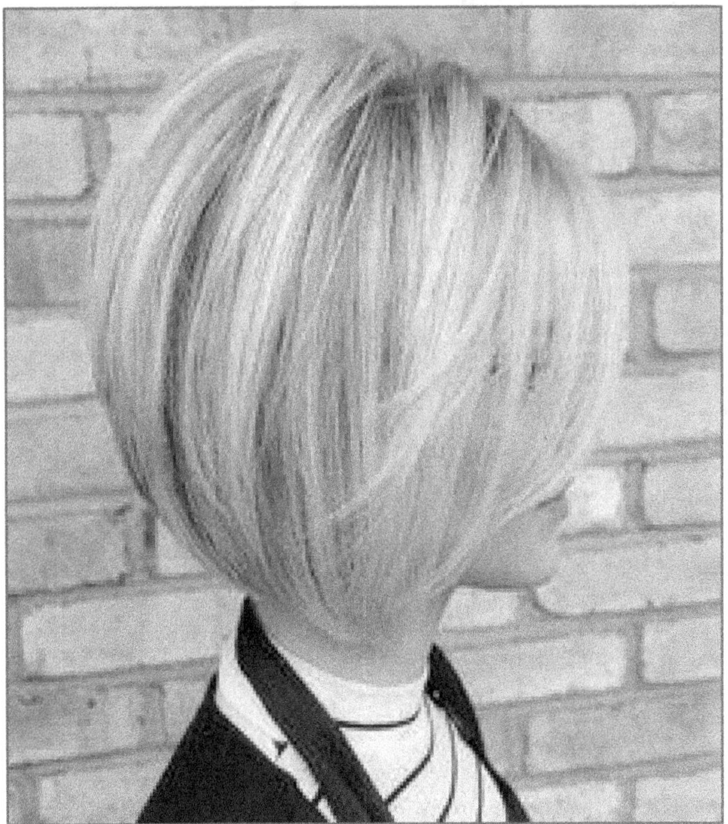

Any blowout is refined, classy, and chic. Use a volumizing mousse right out of the shower to add fullness and combat wispy hair, then blow dry with a round brush. In order to highlight your healthy, luscious hair, finish with a shine spray.

Disconnected Choppy Lob Cut

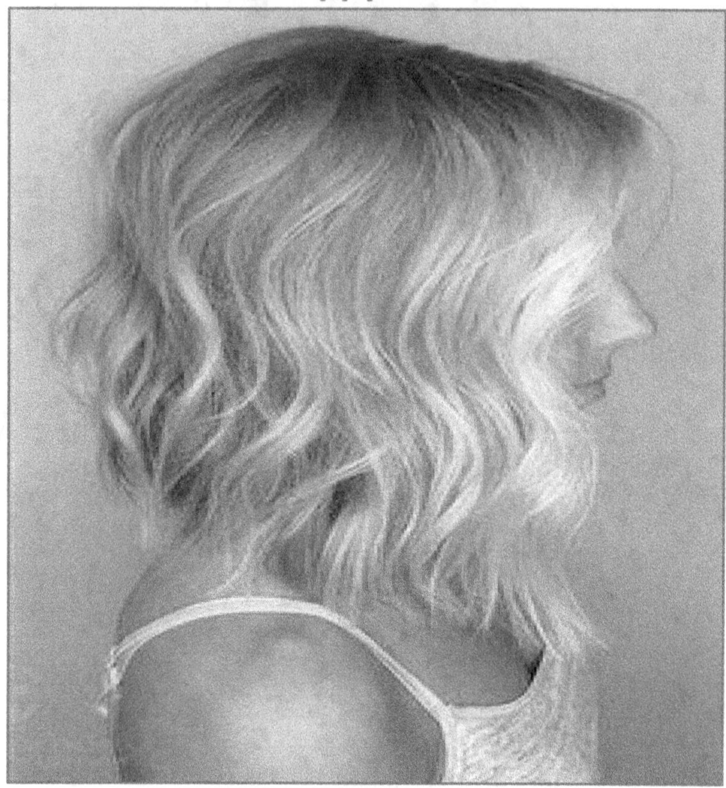

Are you sick of the same old hairstyles for thin fine hair? By literally "twisting" your hair with a flat iron to give them a tiny bend, you may give your unconnected lob a twist. Your dazzling blonde balayage will gain additional fullness and volume if you add some texture to it.

Long Textured Bob with Bronde Balayage

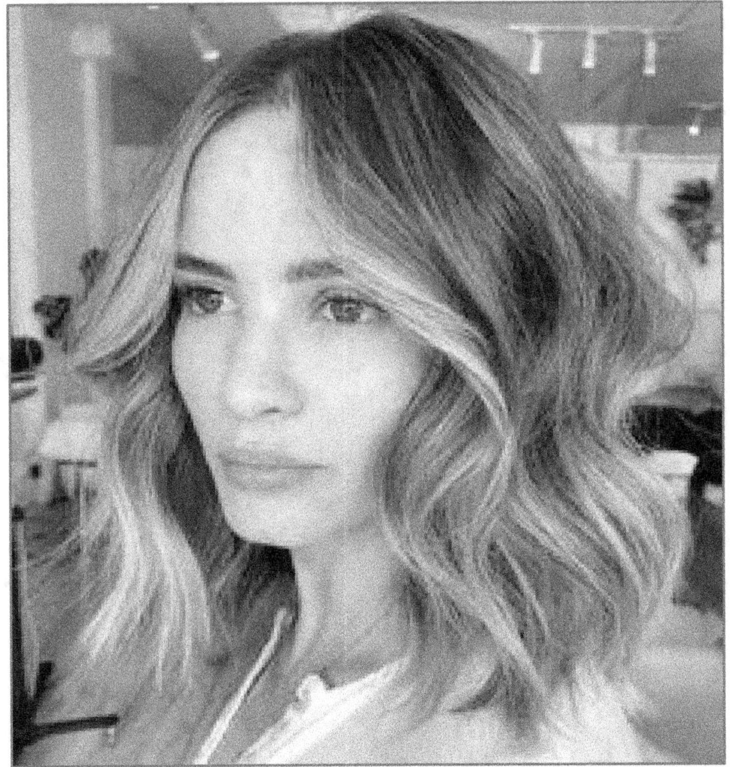

If your hair is on the finer side and straight, shoulder-length locks with a subtly tinted bronde balayage are a timeless style to try. Your face is beautifully framed by the lighter streaks at the front of this long, textured haircut, which also helps to hide the flatness of your hair.

Blonde Haircut with a Shadow Root

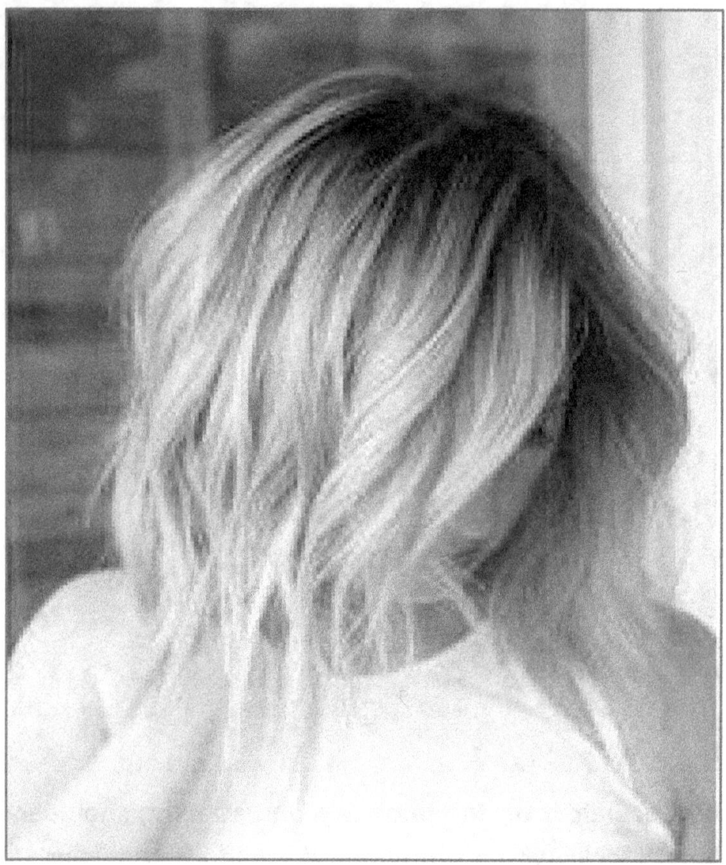

Another instance of a dye job that works well with thin haircuts! In addition to being practical for a boss on a budget, a shadow root also offers the aesthetic depth that fine hair needs.

Gray and Platinum Bob with Chopped Ends

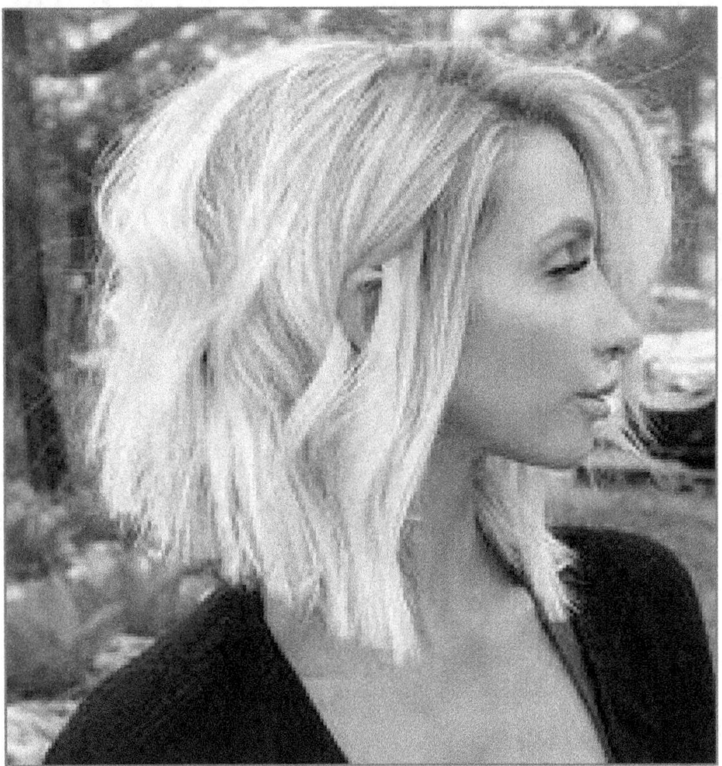

Adding some texture and movement can increase the volume and body of your tresses if you have straight hair. Use a straightener to bend the hair and a brush to run through the strands for a stylish, texturized look.

Choppy blonde Lob

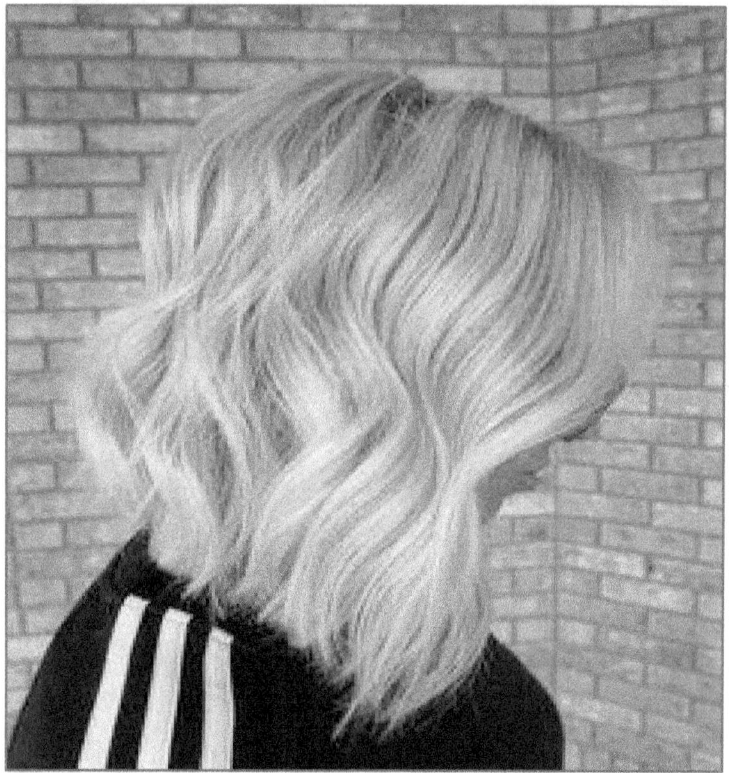

Consider a chopped cut in a medium length if your hair is straight and your stylist doesn't suggest haircuts for thin hair with V-cut layers. A lob is a good alternative. If you are a blonde, go for a delightful hair colour like this creamy blonde balayage, or if you are a brunette, get a colour inspired by rich chocolate delicacies.

Middle Part and Face-Framing Layers

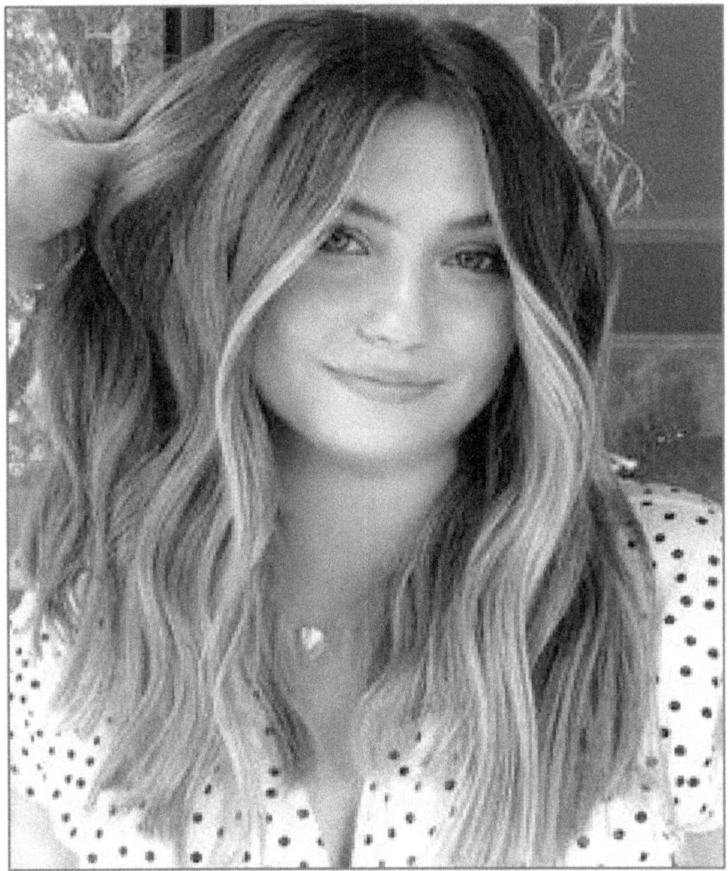

Hairstyles with a centre part enhance oblong and oval faces. Here is a straightforward modern look that features symmetrical framing and big, free waves that are subtly accented with balayage highlights.

Shoulder-Length Shattered Cut with Layers

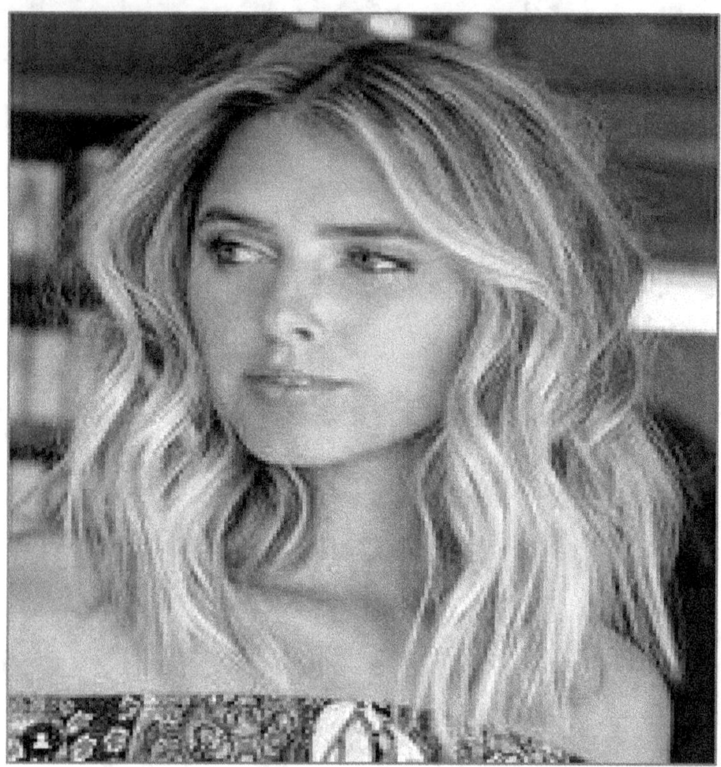

There are numerous hairstyles for thin hair that work with various wave and curl patterns available for those with thin, curly hair. If you want to give your hair a playful and young appearance, think about a golden-blonde balayage.

Blonde Bob with Beach Waves

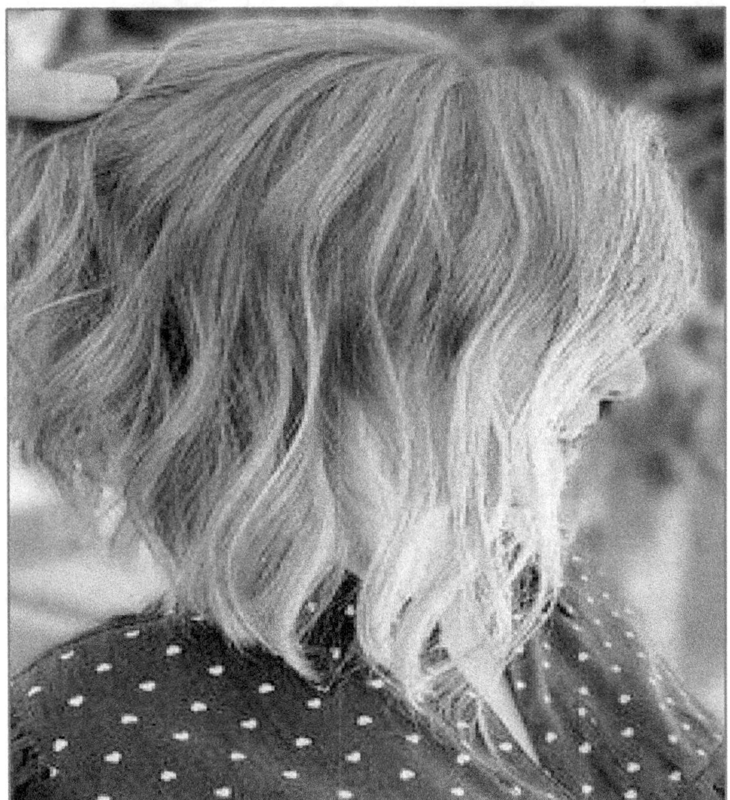

Your best friend for creating volumes styles is texture. This is as simple as letting your naturally wavy, thin hair air dry after washing! For those women with straight hair, consider adding texture by misting damp hair with a homemade sea salt and water solution.

Light Brown and Caramel Balayage

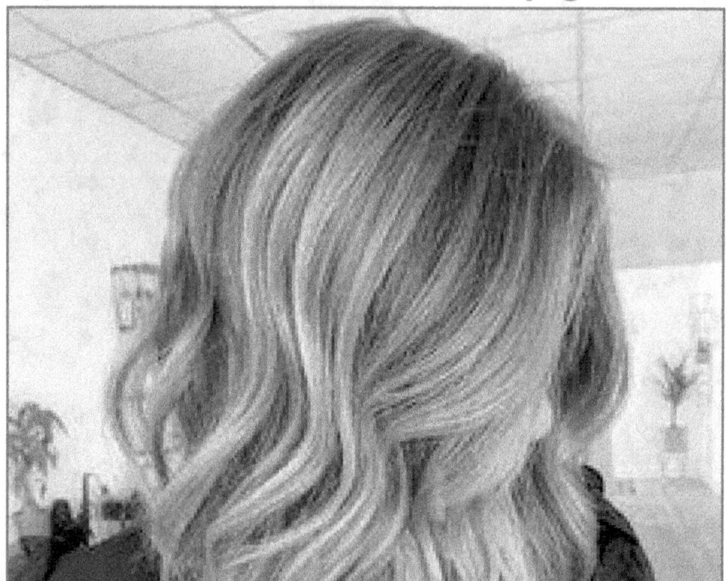

With the help of a gorgeous balayage and shoulder-length layers, show off your inner cool girl. Loose waves that increase the volume of your hair finish off the gorgeous combination. One of the best options to think about if your hair is thin.

Poker-Straight Razored Bob

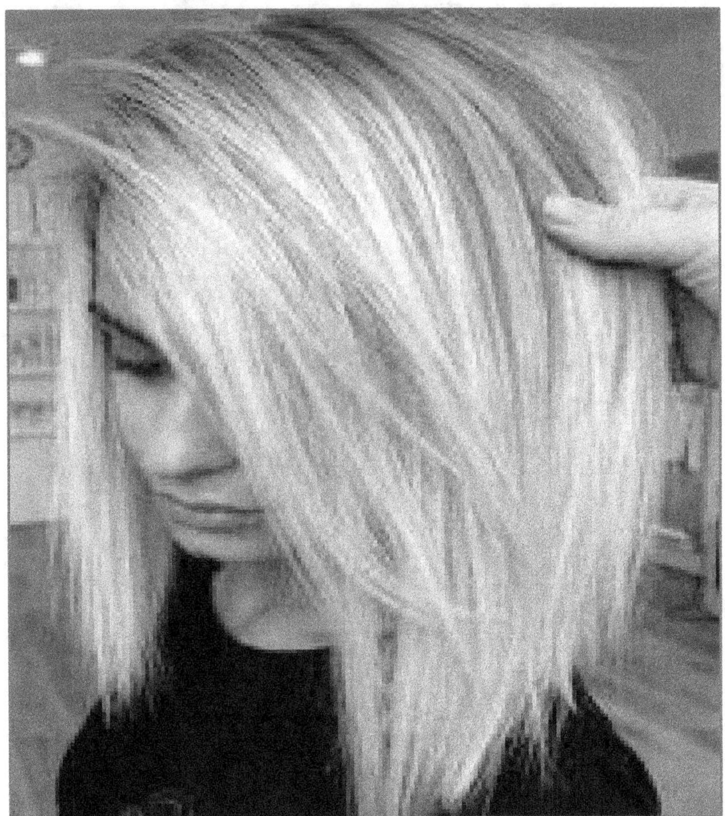

The straight edges of bluntly cut lobs provide the appearance of chunkiness and fullness, making them the ideal hairstyles for thin, fine hair. You can also slightly heighten the top portion by creating a deep side part and flipping the bangs into a combover style.

Mid-Back Cut with Subtle Layers

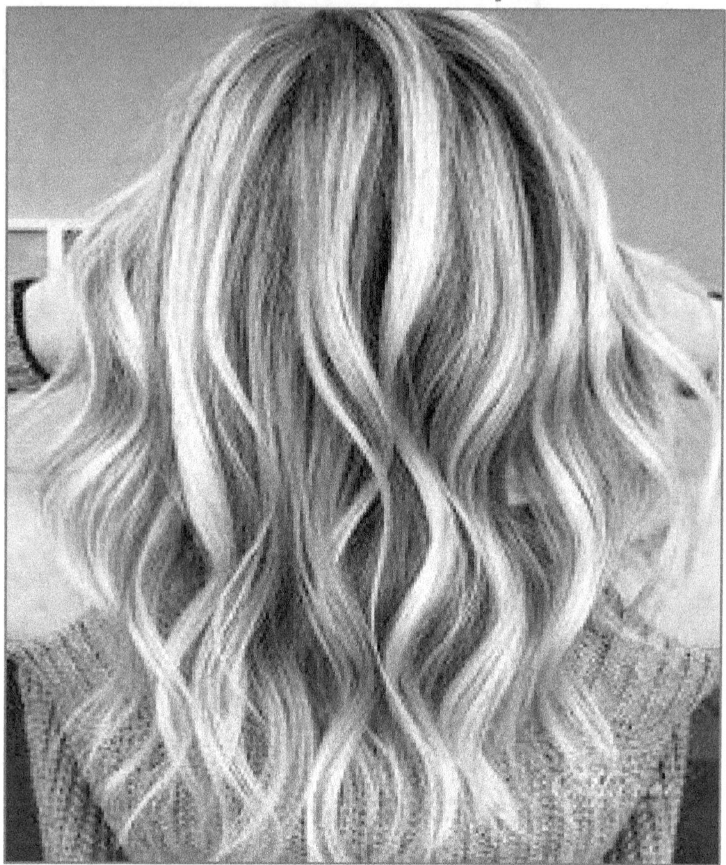

It might be difficult to find hairstyles that offer fullness and depth when you have medium-length locks that are thin. Nevertheless, with dimensional balayage and enough waves, you can easily achieve.

Disconnected White Blonde Lob

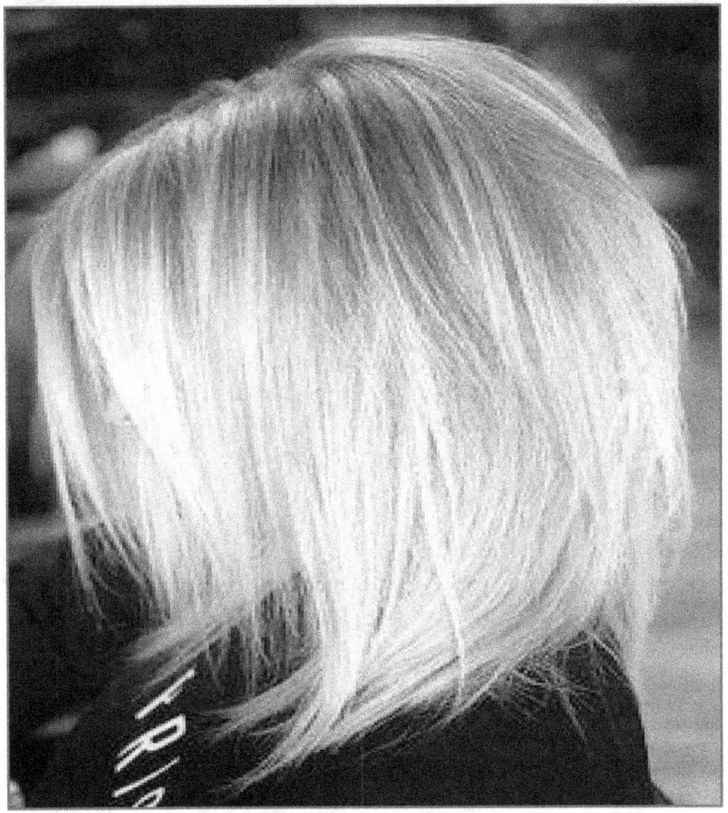

Your fine hair might appear thick and healthy thanks to the long, fluffy lob. Because of how much volume and texture the "disconnected" style creates, it's one of the greatest haircuts for thin hair. For a bold fashion statement, go with a bright white blonde shade.

Sexy Cinnamon Haircut

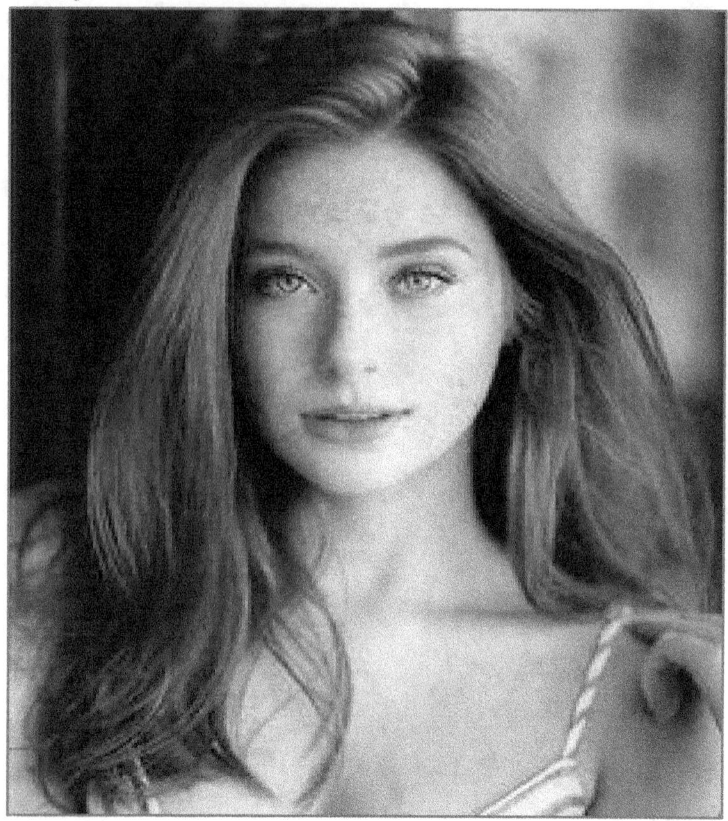

Because it is rich and deep without standing out too much from any scalp that may be seen through sparse strands, reddish brown is an excellent color for thin hair. Make sure to only use light colors as a face-framing element if you want to add them.

Bright Blonde Bob with Shaggy Ends

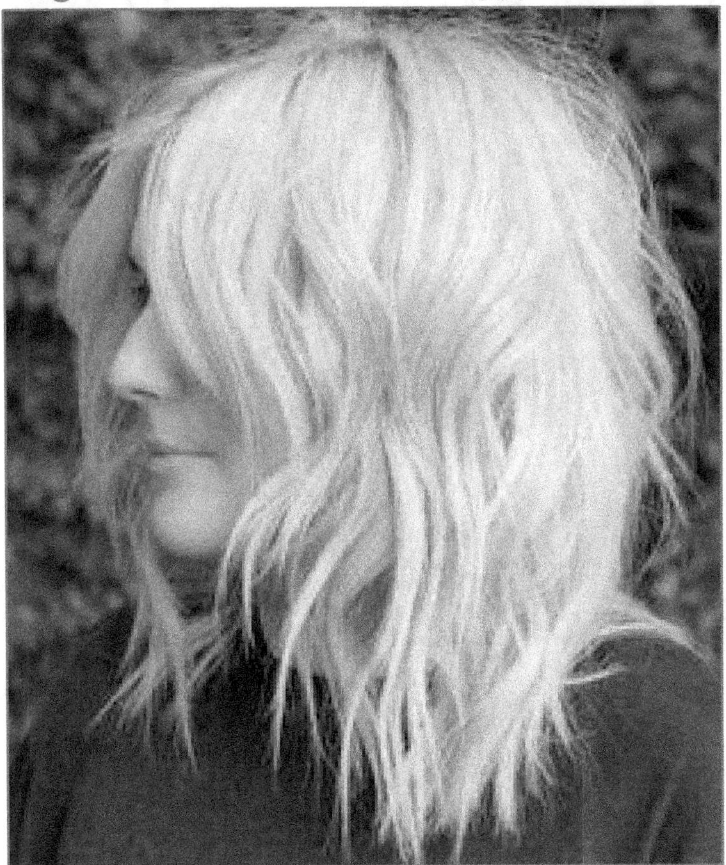

A center-parted, bleached blonde bob shag is the sexiest hairstyle ever. Choppy ends add to the texture's feel and keep your hair looking healthy and shining. White blonde waves contrast well with dark brown roots.

Short Layered Bob Haircut

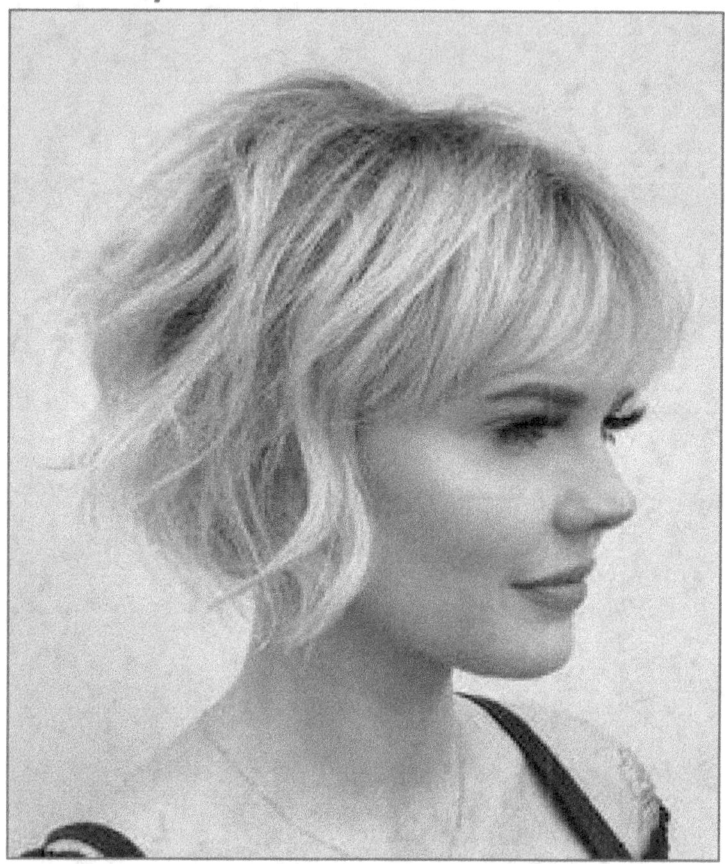

Texture and color are two certain ways to change thin hair. Choppy layers provide volume, while dark roots against light hair instantly create the impression that your strands are dense.

Caramel Balayage on Short Hair

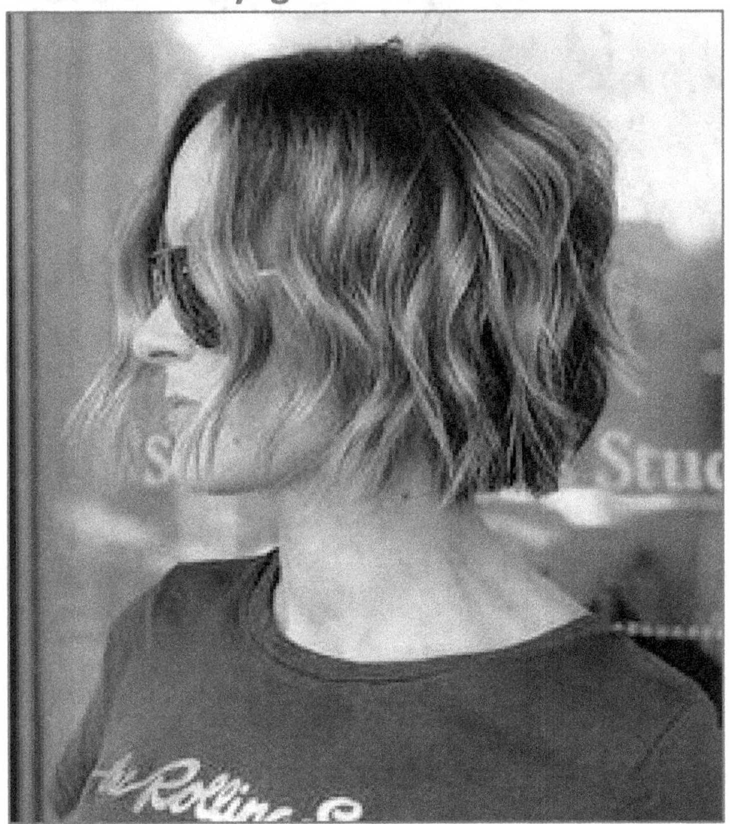

By contrasting your chocolate bob with caramel highlights, you may give your haircut a lovely and sweet look. Make it sweeter by giving it loose curls. This hairdo is suitable for everyday wear and conveys femininity and romance.

Long Layered Haircut with Curtain Bangs

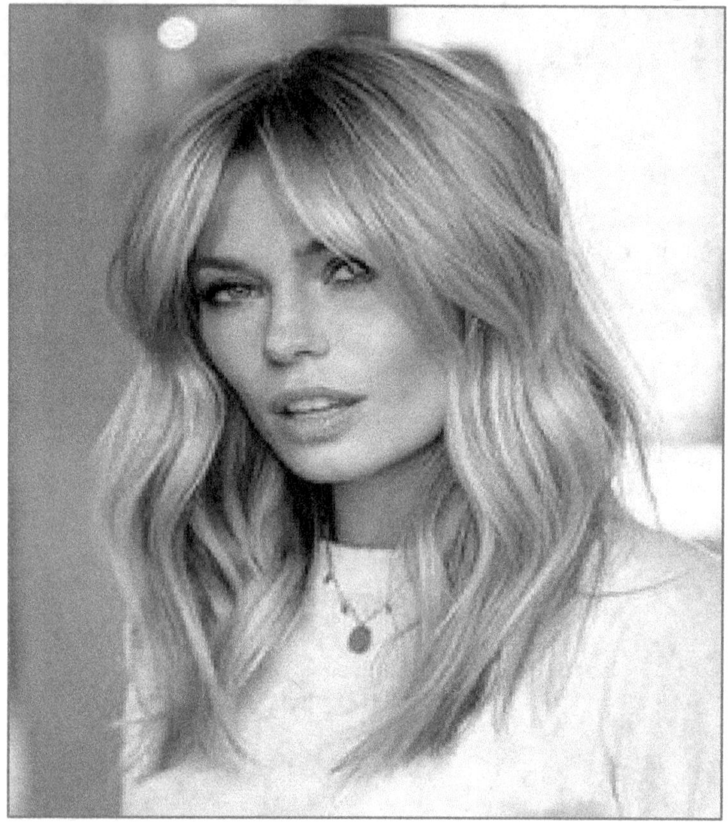

Try the curtain bangs as an easy approach to highlight the volume of your layered cut. These can be effectively used to add the width that narrow haircuts frequently lack.

Brown Lob with Highlights

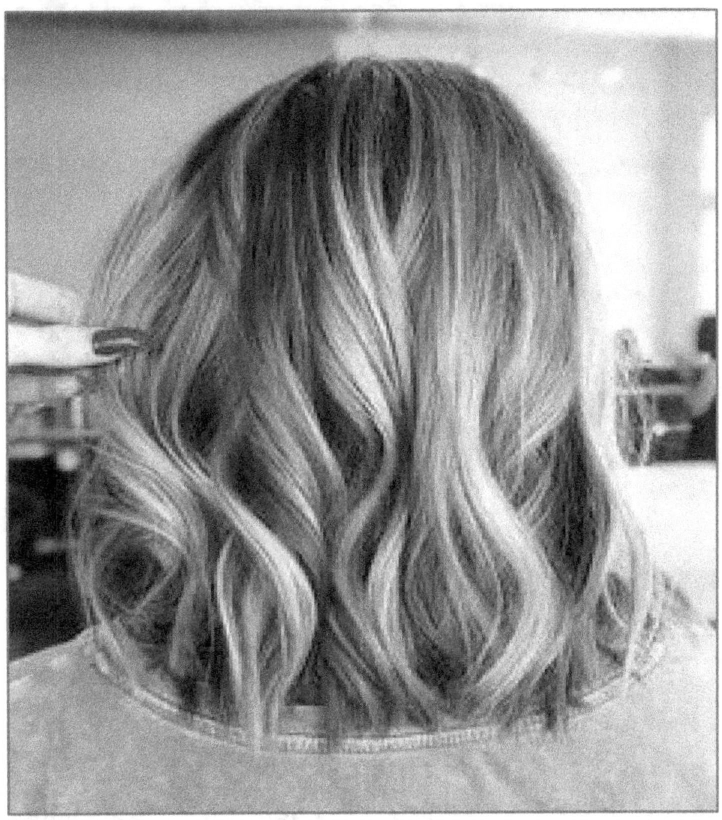

Your fine hair will move more if you give it a light curl and a bend in the ends. The sway and bounce of this bob might be its greatest features. It is what gives the haircut its flirtatious and entertaining qualities while also emphasizing how voluminous your tresses are.

Dusty Pink Shadow Root Bob

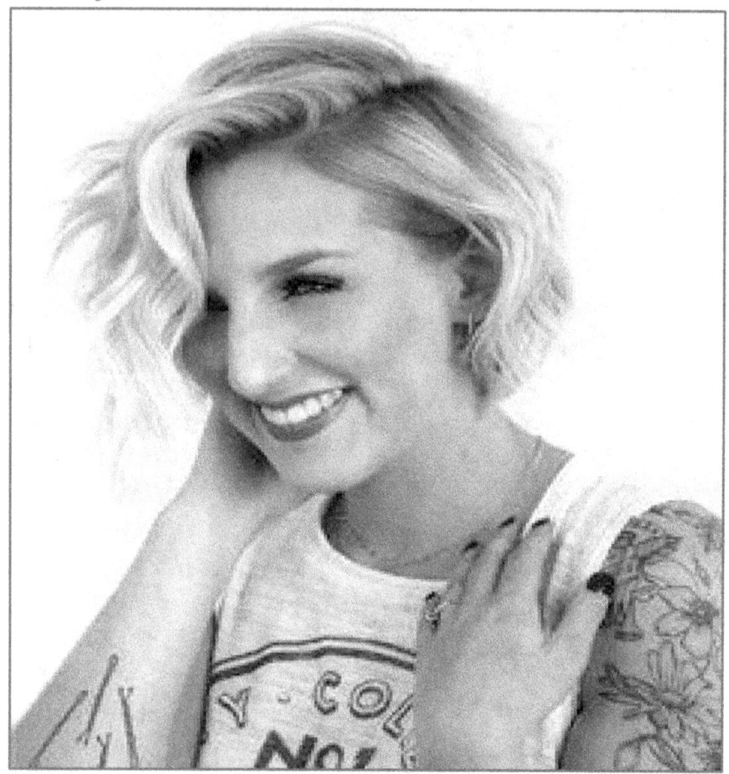

Don't forget to enjoy yourself; let your inner imagination loose and choose a colorful color for your roots! Although the maintenance requirements may be higher, how sick are these dusty pink shadow roots? Liberated from insecurities... When you wear this fashionable look, no one will notice that your hair is thin.

Icy Blonde Layers for Fine Hair

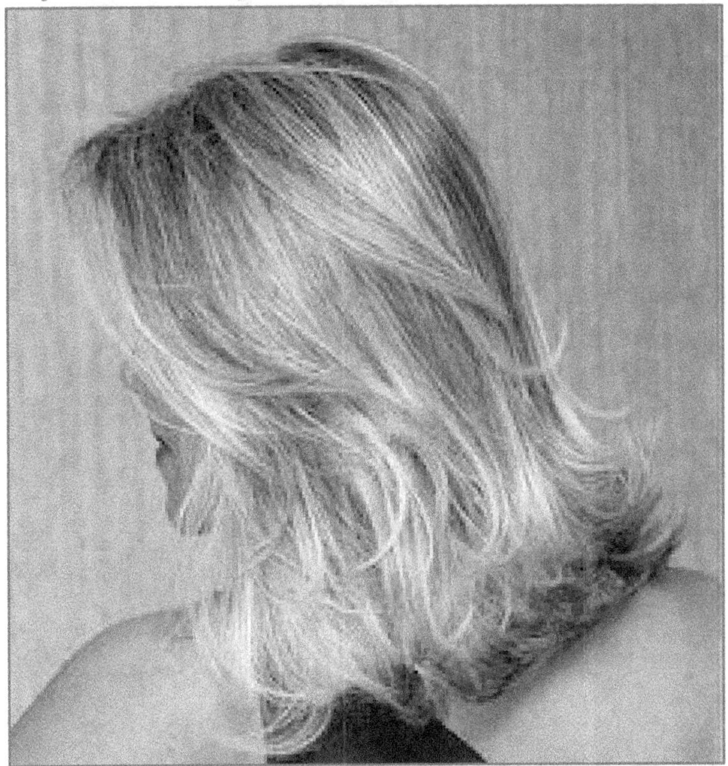

Many older ladies are aware that hair thinning is an unavoidable fact of life. For older women who want to wear longer layered styles and have colder skin tones, here is a great ice blonde option.

Chocolate and Caramel Wavy Lob

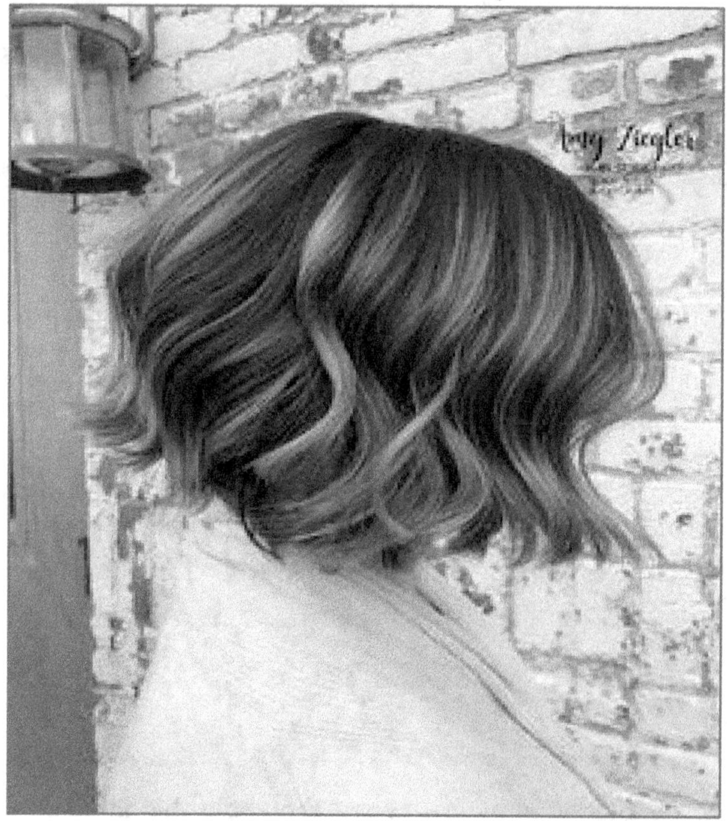

Use some large rollers to create dramatic curves when you want your flat hair to appear thicker. A feeling of fullness and body will be produced by the natural curls and curves. The chocolate base with caramel waves on top looks as delicious as an ice cream sundae!

Beige Bronde Shaggy Lob

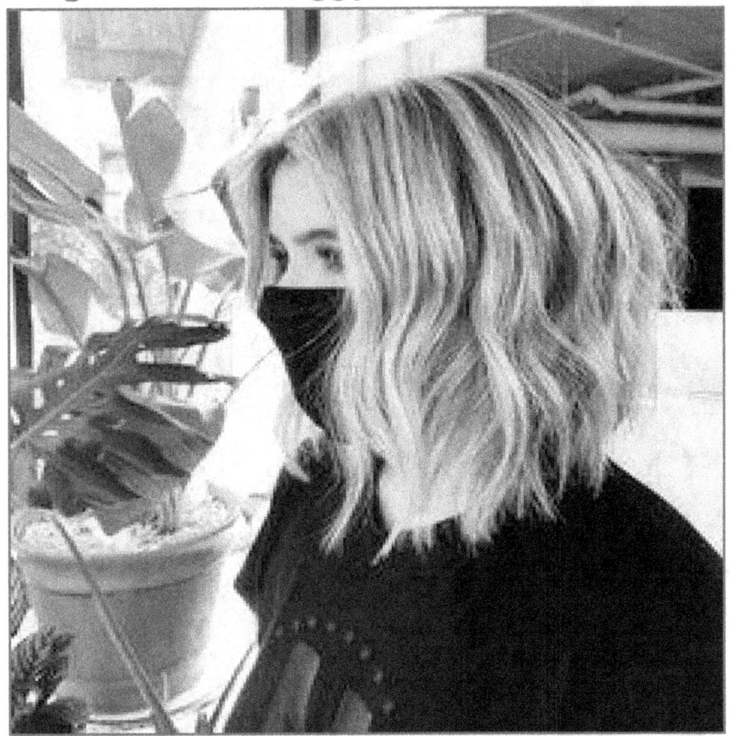

The most common hairstyles for thin-haired ladies today are shoulder-length cuts with a side part. They function much better when the ends are slanted so that the longer portions fall toward the front and when they are little scruffy. The desired depth is added by painting a light beige blonde color over a dark brown background.

Short Shaggy Cut with Textured Ends

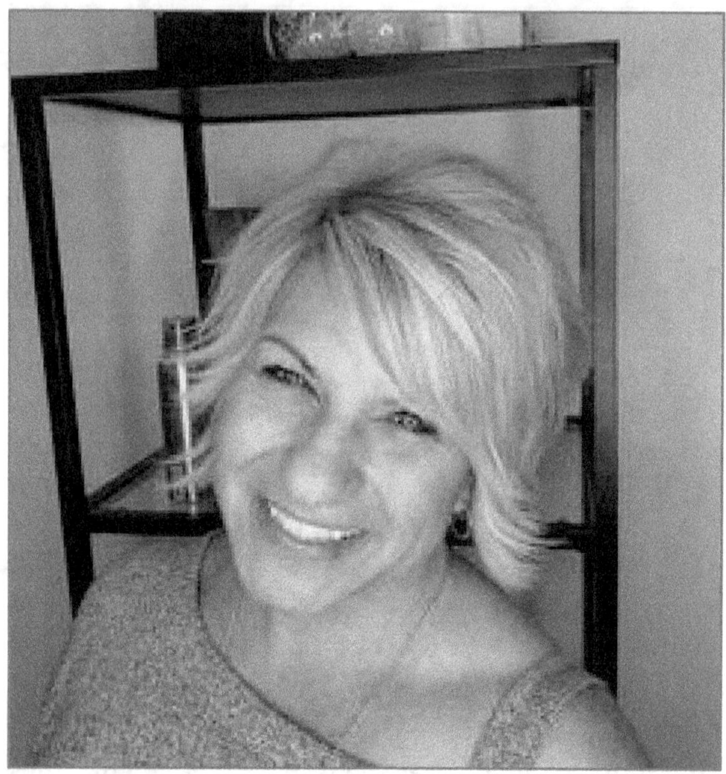

This haircut, like Goldilocks, falls just right in the middle between a bob and a pixie. This haircut avoids seeming flat because to the expertly applied layers that give it a fluffy, feathery appearance.

Cute Layered Haircut for Thin Hair

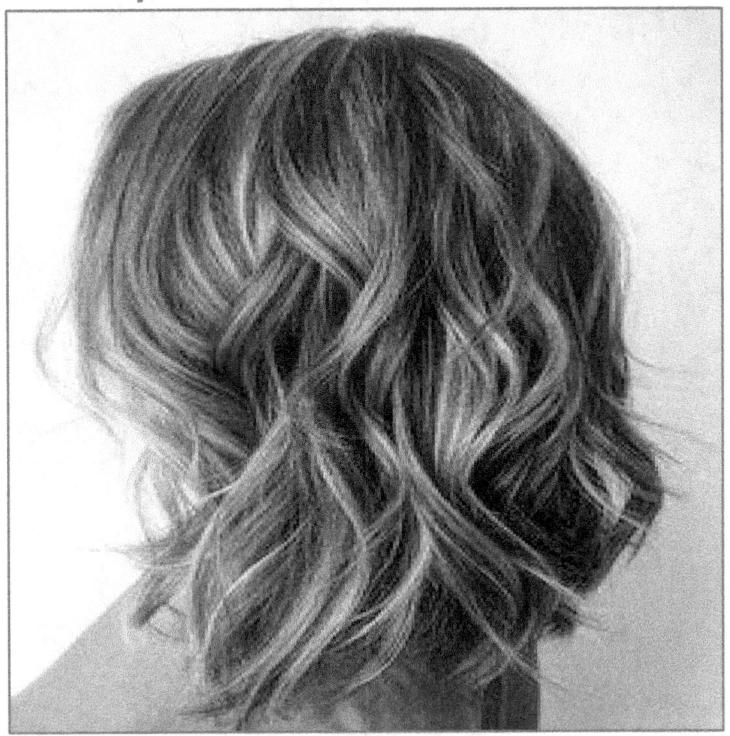

Messy waves complement highlighted hair the best because they offer interest to a typical style. The gorgeous contrast between the lighter blonde at the front and the darker brown down the lower layers makes thin hair appear thicker. The perfect color scheme for the warmer months is provided by these lovely tones.

Short Haircut with Long Fringe

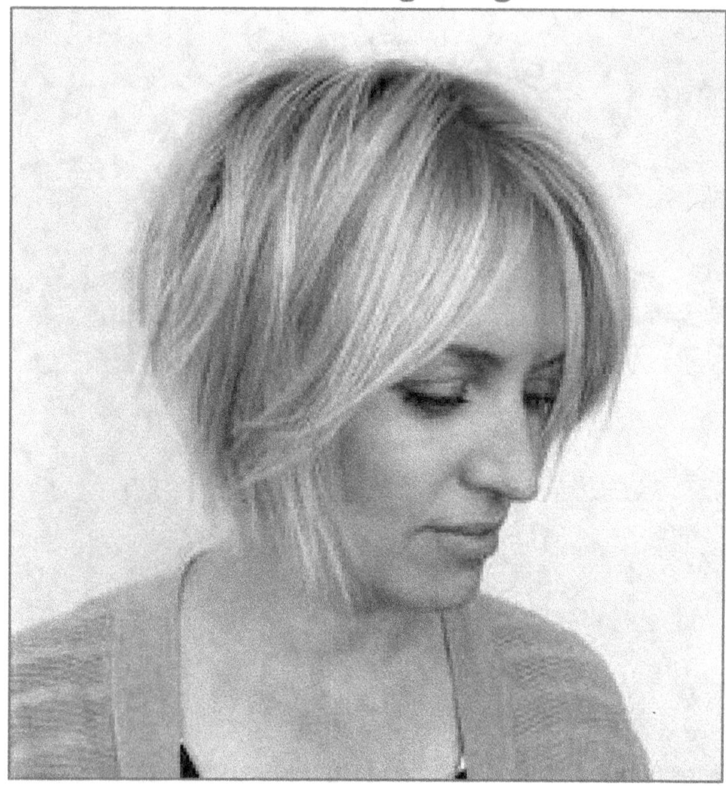

A short, layered cut that tapers at the nape of your neck is a tried-and-true method hairstylists employ on fine hair, whether it is styled straight or curly. Keep a long fringe as a face framing if chops seem scary.

Short Hair with Deep Side Part

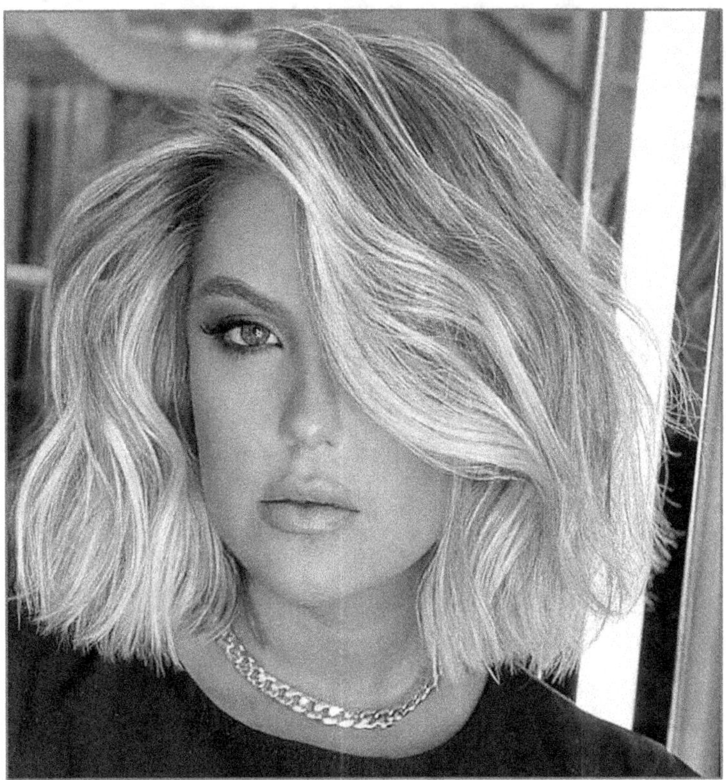

Sometimes changing just the part may give your hair the appearance of thickness! To give exquisite manes the appearance of denseness, rock side bangs with a deep side part. With thin, short hair, this approach works very well. Layering around the crown wisely is also very beneficial.

Medium Length and Wavy Texture

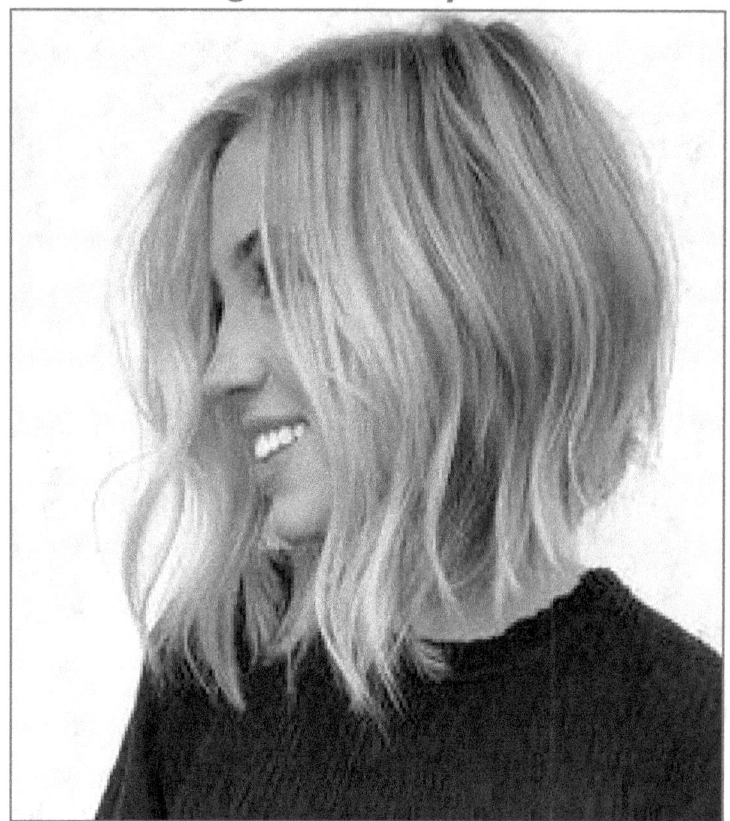

Big waves arranged in midi-length hair have a really romantic appeal. After using a straightening or curling iron, flip your hair around and tousle the waves for more volume, or tease the roots to make the style appear less "done".

Side-Swept Bob

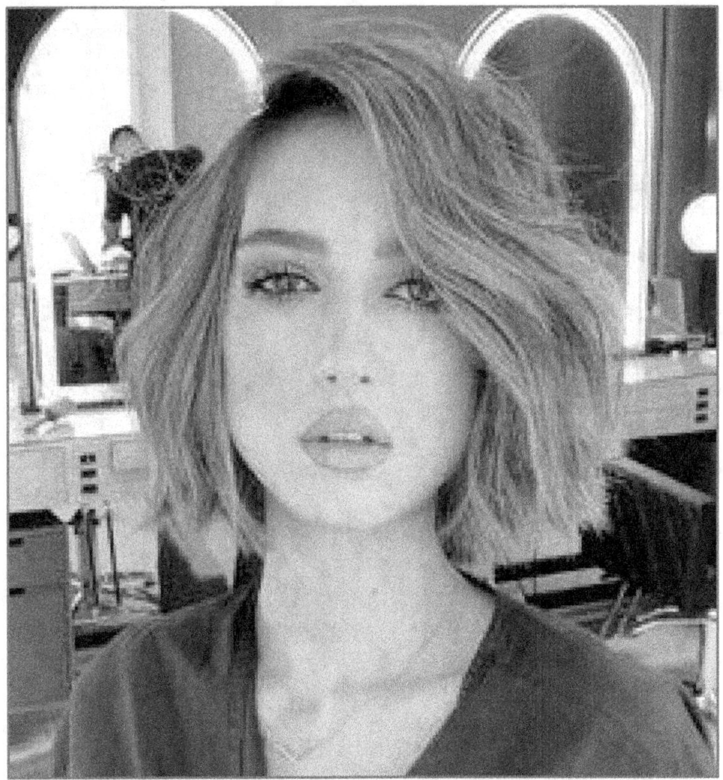

Consider universal cuts like bobs or pixies. Some haircuts for thin hair are very similar to haircuts for thick hair. Although they do vary in appearance depending on the woman's hair type, blowouts are also universally appealing and unquestionably improve the volume and smoothness of short hair.

Thin Chopped Shag

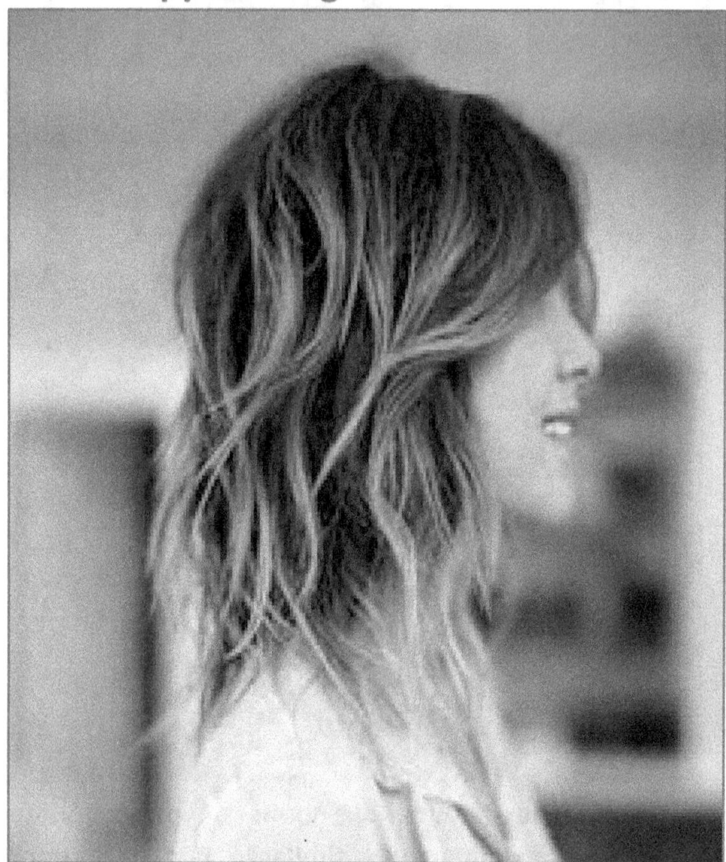

This is a contemporary interpretation of the shag. It looks modern and fresh thanks to the choppiness, and the layering adds some much-needed body. For any woman with thinning hair, this gorgeous mid-length cut is ideal.

Long Bob with Layers

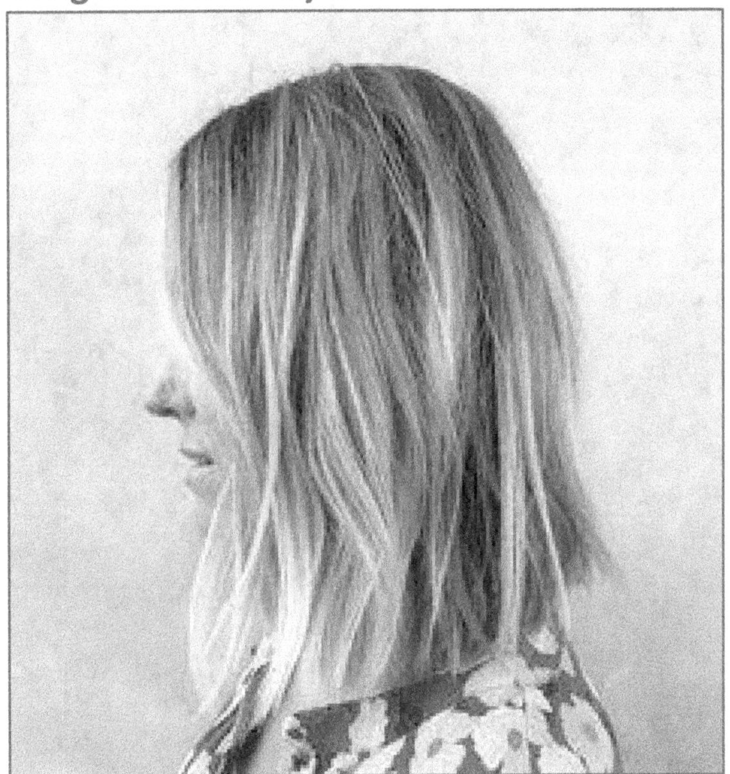

Layers are used to add extra body to hairstyles for women with thin hair. Even on your busiest days, the variety of lengths in your hair prevent it from seeming lifeless. You can leave the house quickly in the morning without damaging your hair with a quick wash and go and some hair serum.

Angled Lob with Bright Blonde Balayage

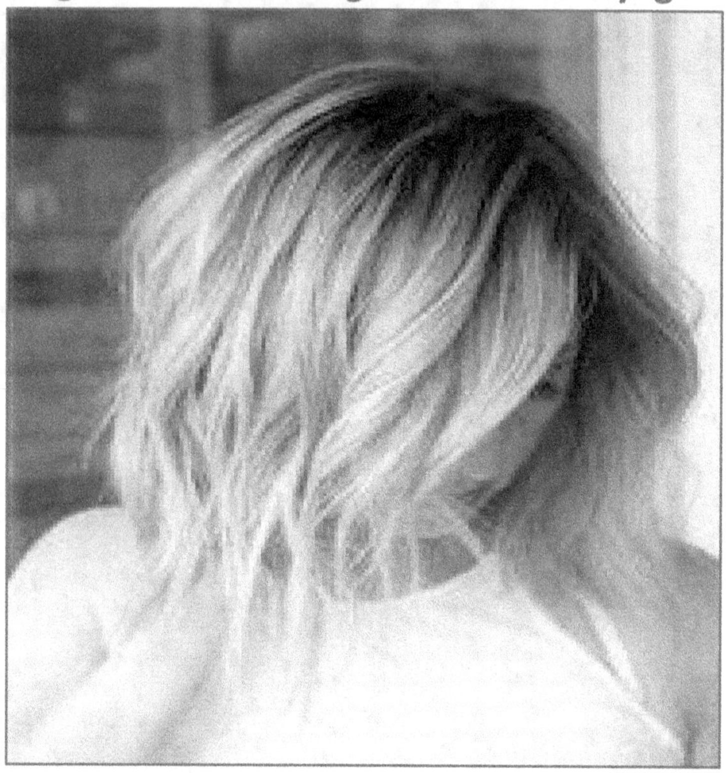

The long bob, or "lob," is a relatively recent variation on the traditional bob. Thanks to its little layering and asymmetry, this cut checks all the boxes if you're looking for a good haircut to make thin hair look thicker. Consider adding a balayage or babylights to boost the look.

Long A-Line Bob

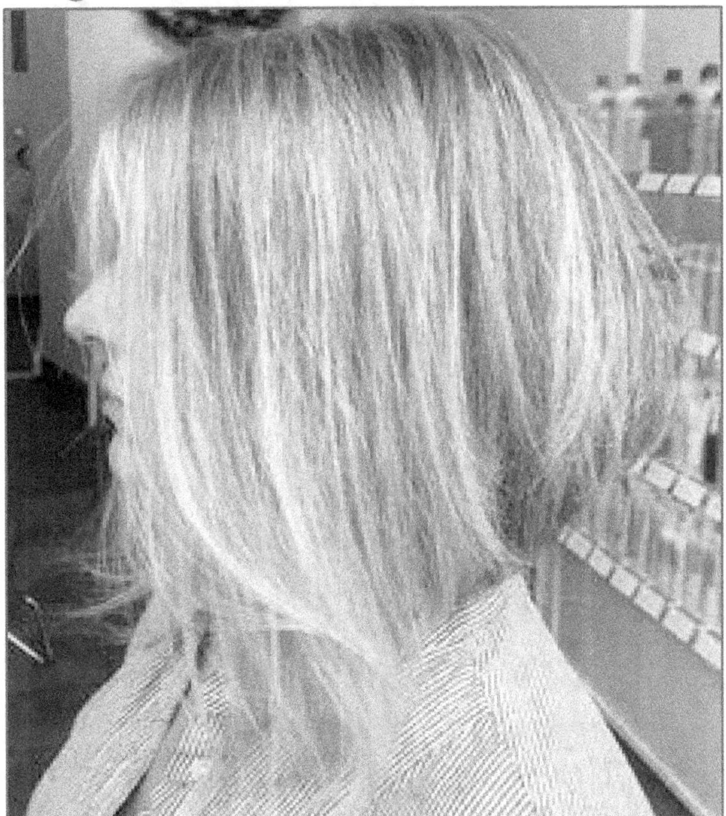

Not all women prefer layers, and single-length haircuts are making a great comeback. A long a-line bob's regularity gives thinner hair a contemporary look. Don't worry about having to run to the salon frequently; this cut also looks fantastic when it has grown out.

Layered Honey and Platinum Hairstyle

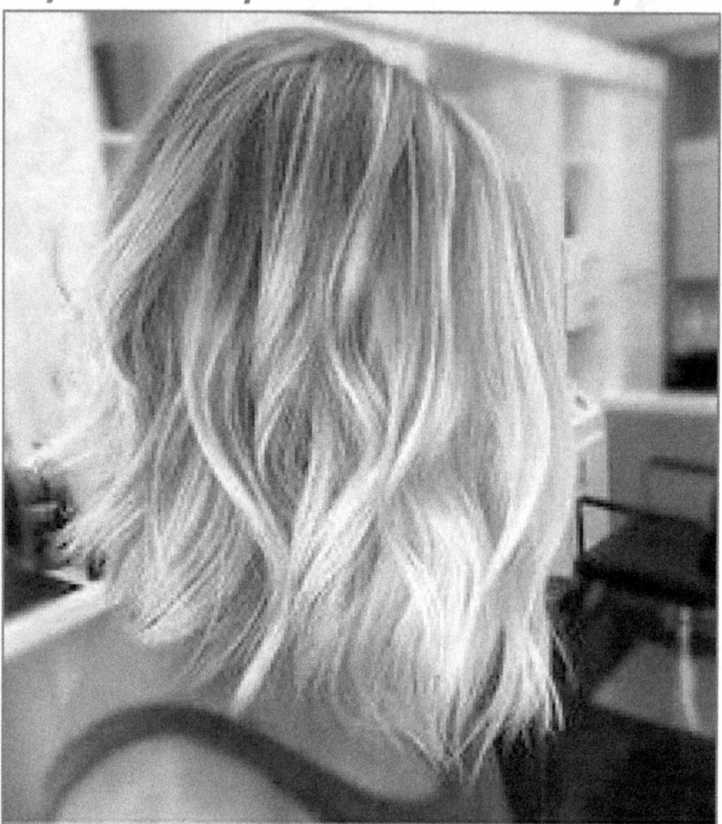

The best haircuts for ladies with thin hair are those with layers. Hair looks fuller when the length of the tresses varies. An easy solution is to simply add more layers to the cut you are already sporting to make your hair appear thicker.

Voluminous Bob Haircut for Thin Hair with Side Bang

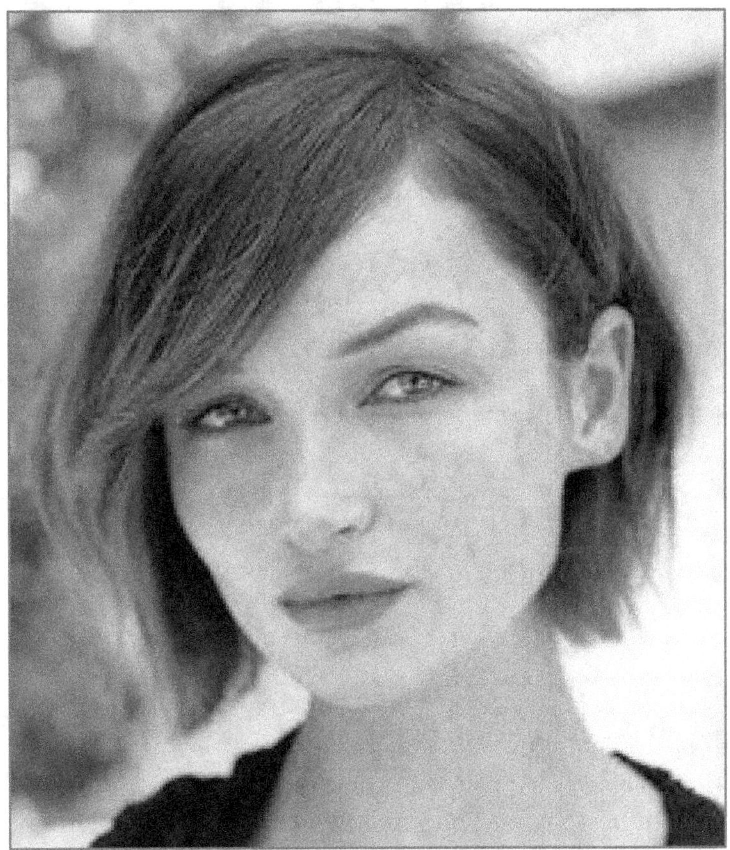

A beautiful hairstyle that can go with any daytime plans you have is a voluminous bob. Wearing the traditional look is equally at home on a date or while running errands.

Long Brown A-Line Bob with Balayage

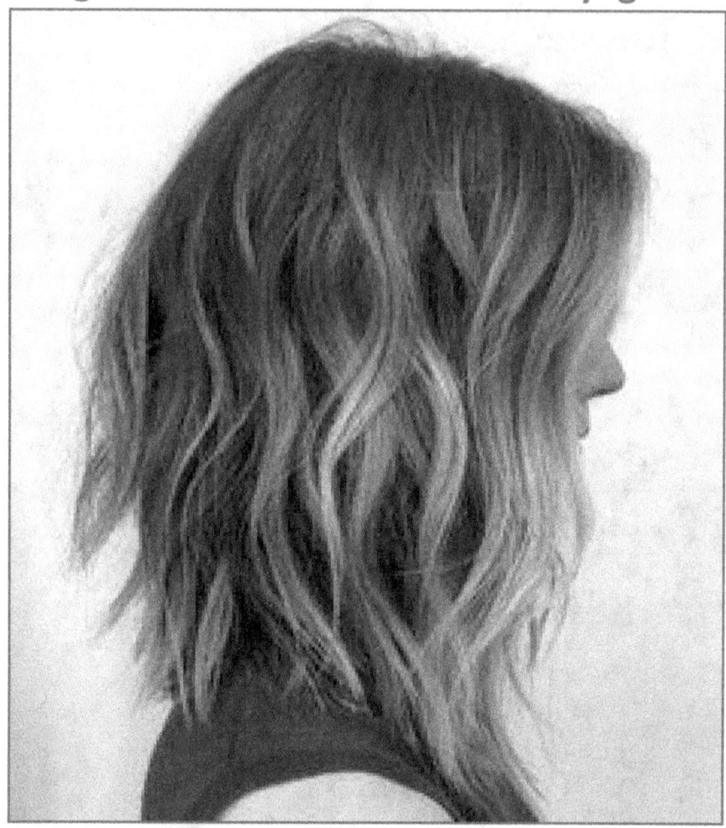

Hairstyles with lots of layers and texture look good on thin hair. To give your hair weight and a delightfully messy look, tousle your fine strands. Shorter hair is easier to manage than long hair, but an angled choppy bob will make a stronger statement.

Stacked Bob for Thin Hair

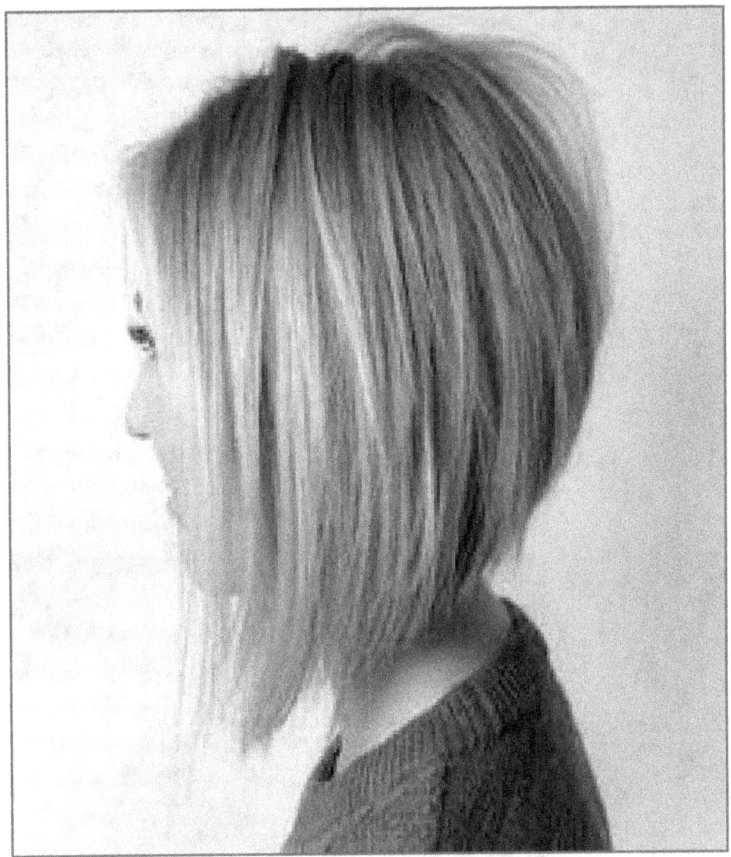

For thin hair, stacked bobs are a traditional haircut. Your nape of the neck has the shortest hair, which instantly adds volume and aesthetic intrigue to the crown of your head.

Messy and Shaggy Haircut for Fine Hair

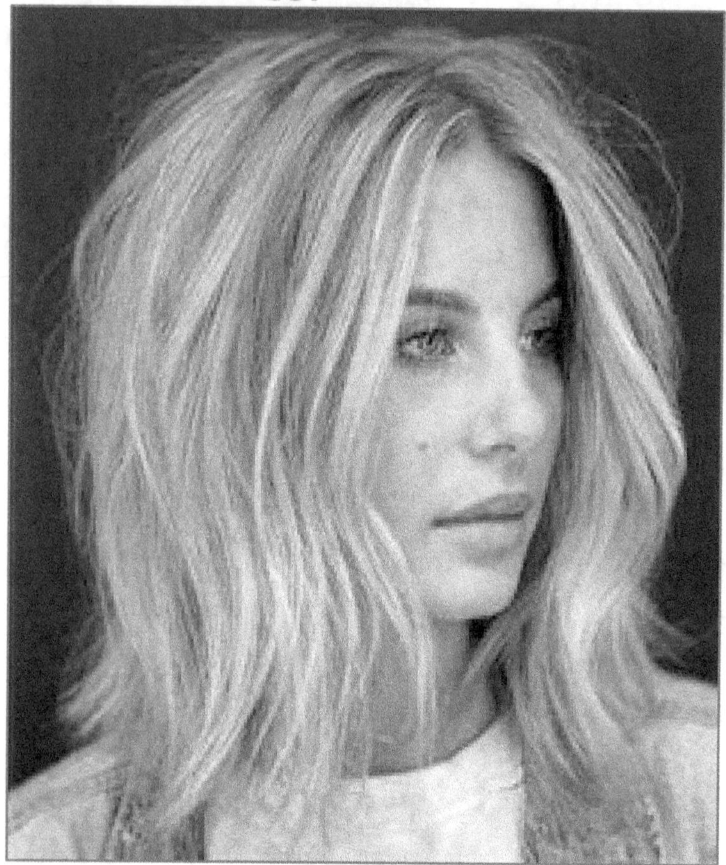

Recall our discussion on texture? Shaggy haircuts are a great way to make the most of razors. This cut has a messy-chic appearance when worn with the appropriate attire and looks fantastic on thin manes.

Strawberry Blonde Bob

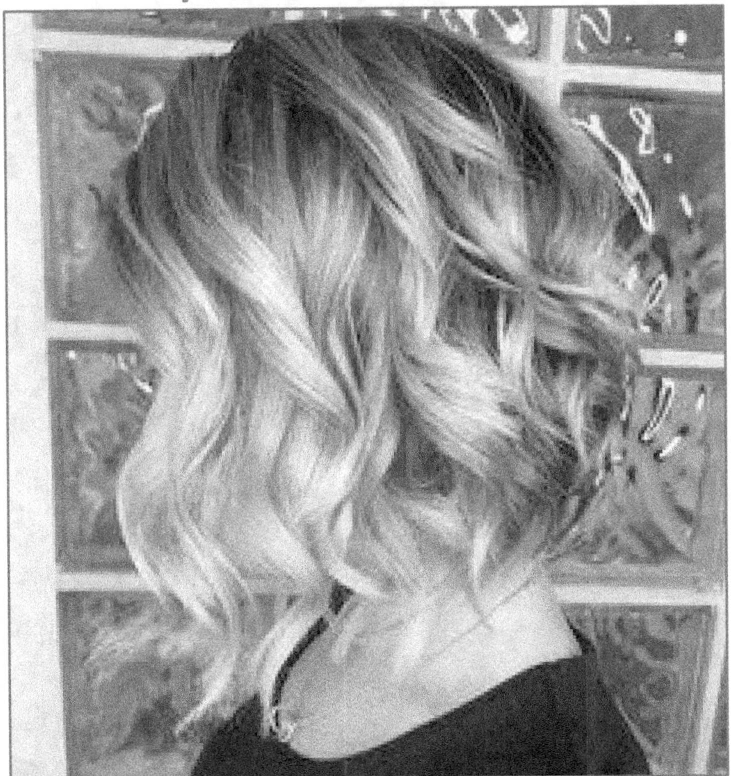

Give your hair a combination of highs and lows if you want to make it appear fuller. The clashing colors that are tangled throughout your hair give you the entire effect you desire. This technique will work on anyone with any hair color, whether they are a rich brunette or a sweet strawberry blonde.

Choppy Dishevelled Lob Hairstyle

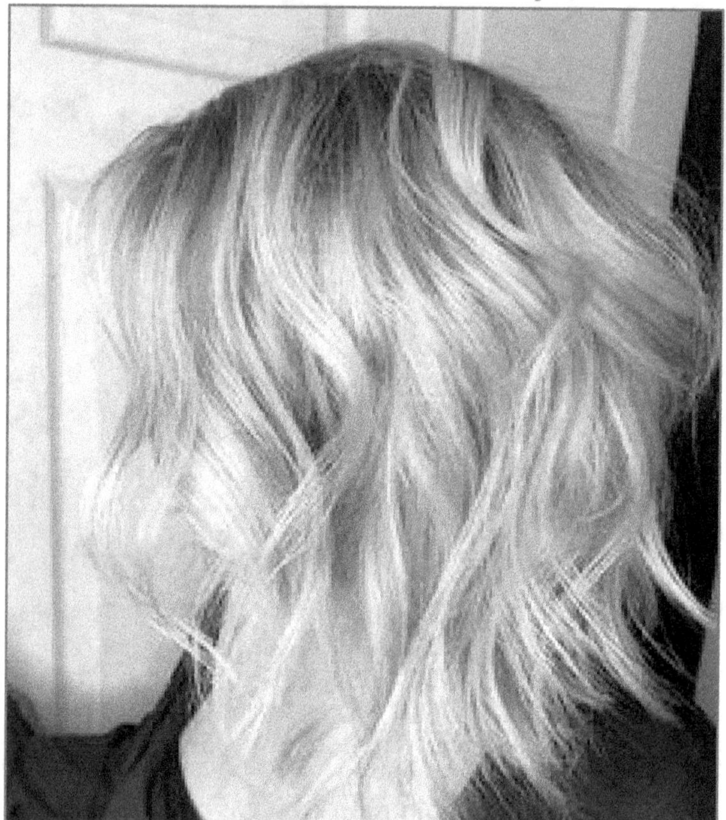

Taking "I woke up like this" a step farther! Although single length cuts are doable, layering is a surefire strategy to use on thin hair. For elegant, successful women, choppy lob hairstyles above the shoulder are quite wonderful options.

Medium Wavy Haircut for Thin Hair

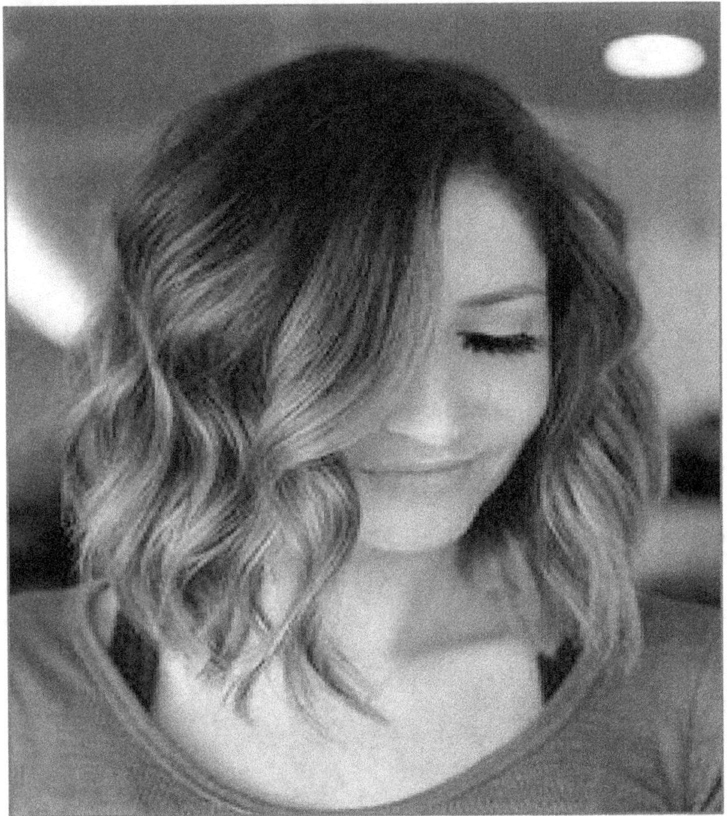

For medium single length haircuts, there are a ton of styling possibilities! The body and movement that curling wands produce are beneficial for thin locks. You may also easily incorporate cute, fast waves with hot rollers into your morning regimen.

Medium Choppy Cut with Long Bangs

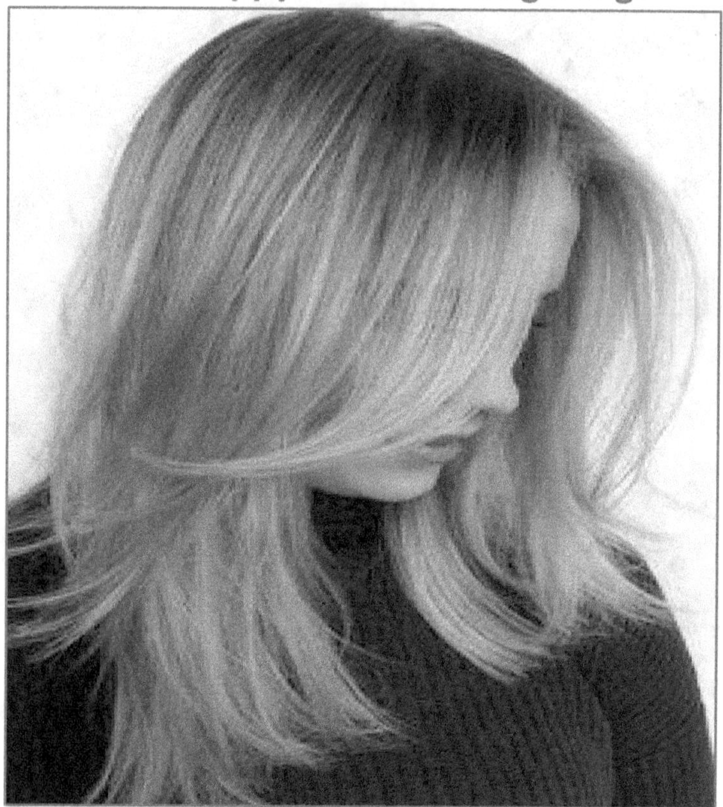

You prefer a flat iron to a curling iron. If long hairstyles for thin hair are trimmed jagged, with strands of various lengths, they will look voluminous when straightened.

Choppy Bob with Blonde Highlights

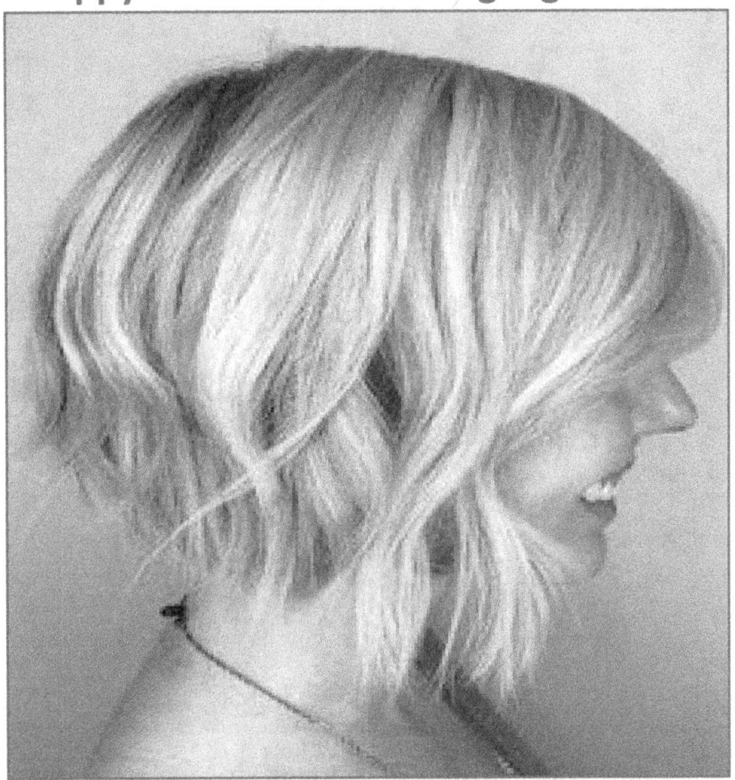

Haircuts for fine, thin hair are quite straightforward, but they look good when done correctly. The best styling tip for a choppy cut is to begin root-to-end tease your hair. The best results come from using a fine-tooth comb. After that, gently shake your hair with your fingers. After you've achieved the ideal sloppy appearance, spray some hairspray with a light hold.

Layered Bob Haircut for Fine Hair

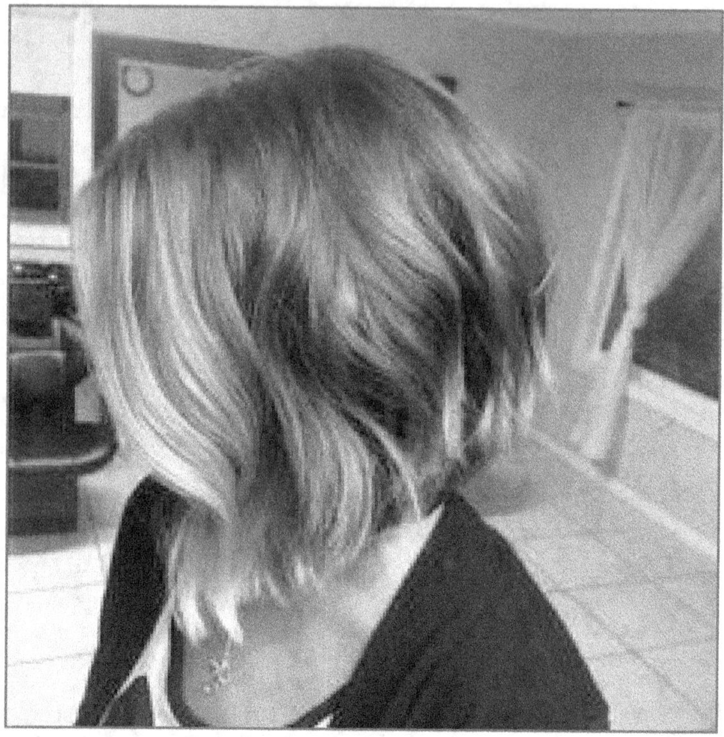

Long hair with substance and gloss is lovely, yet long thin hair can still be lovely. No matter what, women shouldn't aim for longer length. Thin hair can actually look thicker and more lovely when styled in chic, modern bobs with jagged ends and exquisite balayages. Additionally, contemporary short haircuts for thin hair are never dull!

Shattered Collarbone Bob

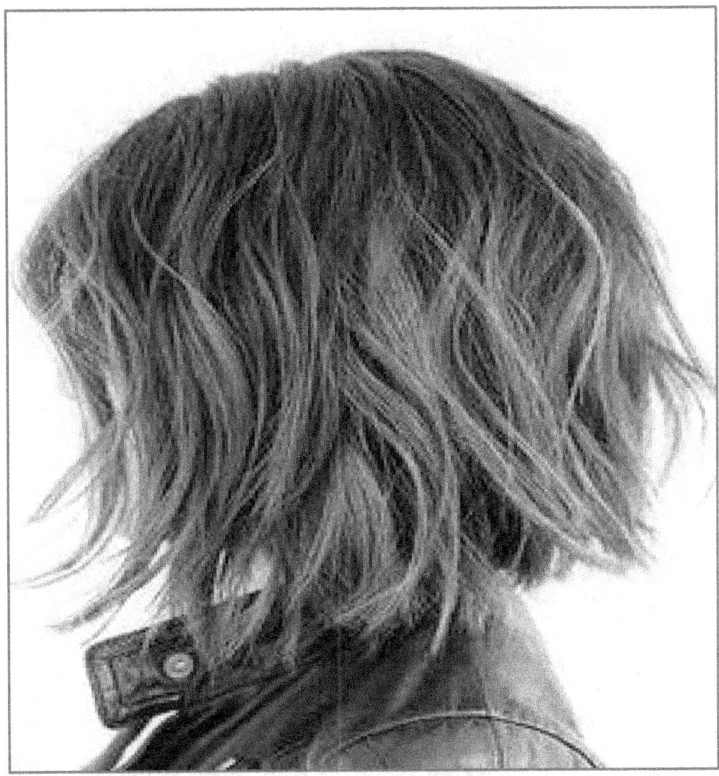

If your hair is thin, a stylish collarbone bob with shattered texture will give it the needed body. The distinctive charming disarray is totally in the spirit of the most popular messy hairstyles of the current season and is created by light layering closer to the edges and A-line side bangs.

Wavy Bob with Layers

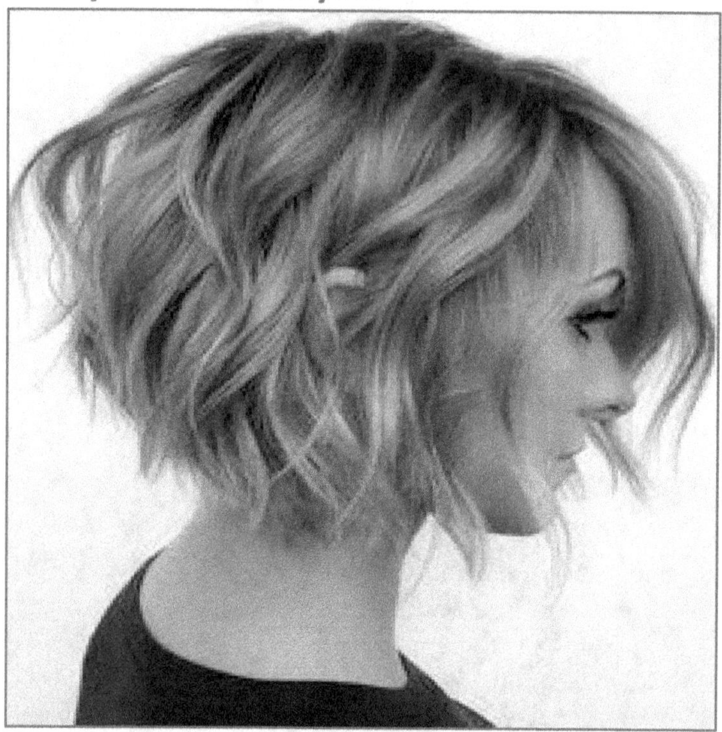

The greatest hairstyles for thin hair sometimes end up being one-length bobs since they give the appearance of thickness. The hair strands lay comfortably on top of one another when the texture is improved, giving the appearance of added fullness. Small introductions of highlights add dimension, which gives the hair depth.

Brunette V Cut for Thick Straight Hair

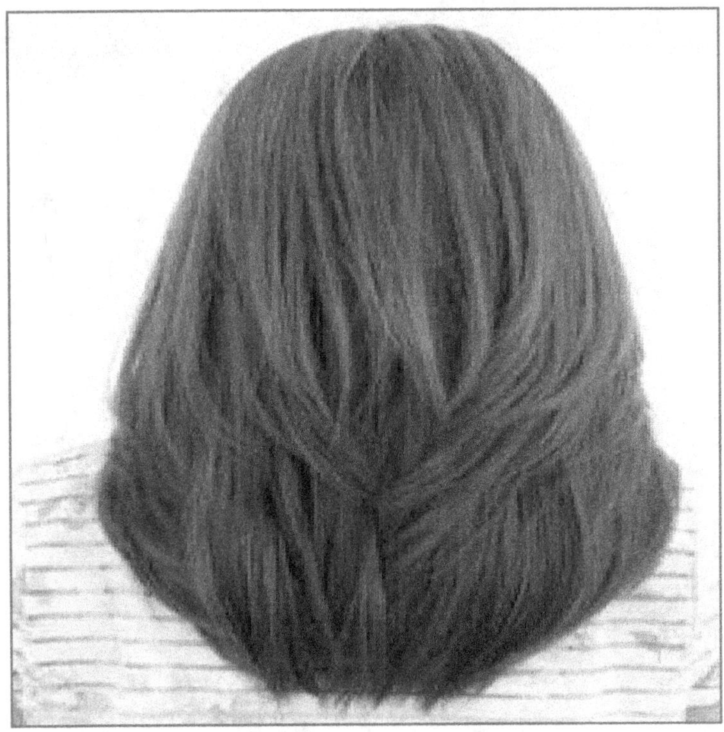

If you have long, thick, straight hair, there's no need to overcomplicate your hair style. Simply shape it into a V with two or three simple layers rather than chopping it into waves or bright highlights. This will make it easier to style with a blow dryer and need less upkeep while also adding texture, symmetry, and aesthetic appeal.

Layered Cut for Long Fine Hair

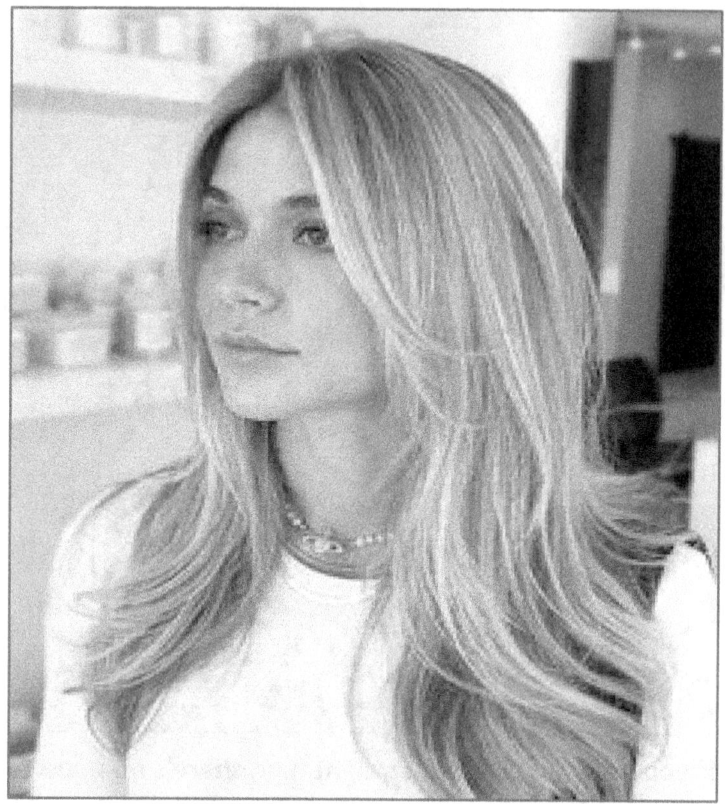

Your naturally dark roots will be enhanced by adding long, feathery layers with blonde highlights to give your long layered hair a beachy feel. The summery colour combination gives your hair a feeling of depth and fullness all throughout, and it seems glossy and sun-kissed. The appearance is finished off by the feathery, fluffy ends.

Very Long Feathered U Cut

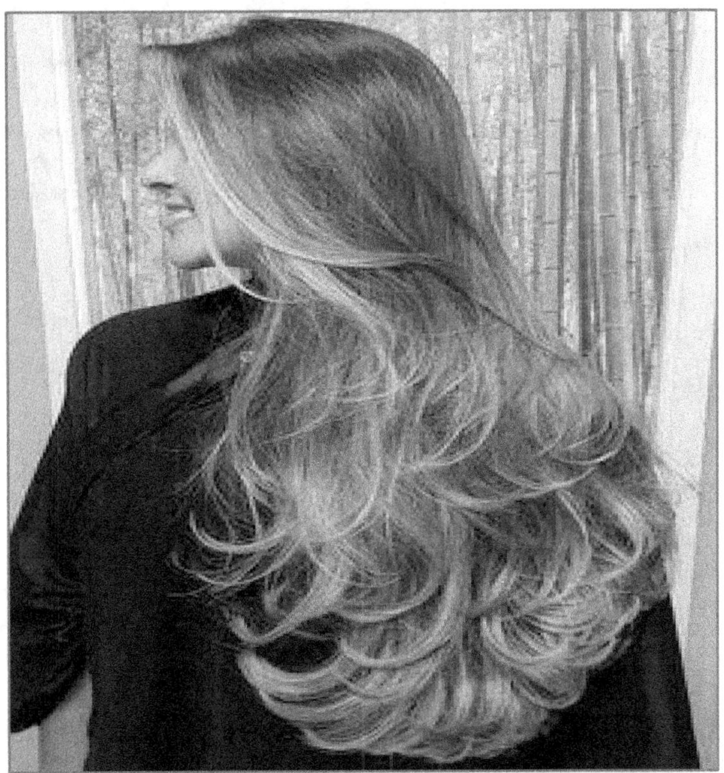

Having long, straight hair is unquestionably one of your greatest accomplishments. Imagine how extra-long hair with gentle feathery layers might look in a free-flowing hairdo! We suggest boosting your hair with a blonde balayage that also lightens your complexion if you have long enough, thick hair to get a similar effect.

Messy Cut with Randomly Chopped Layers

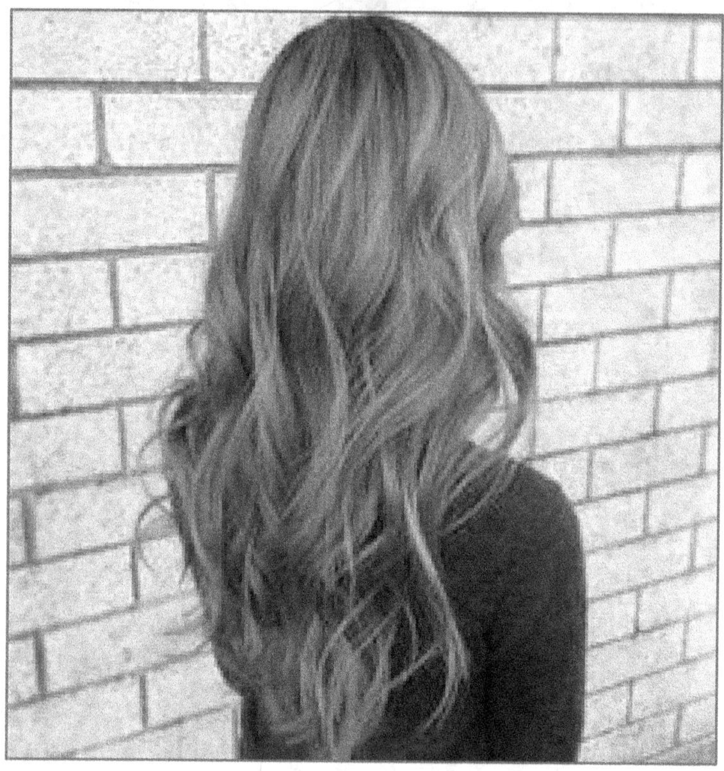

Do you find "organized chaos" appealing? Your hair will reflect that casual attitude if it has randomly cut layers. By arranging it in loose curls or waves that vary in direction, you may prevent hair from seeming stringy.

Light Layers Enhanced by Colour

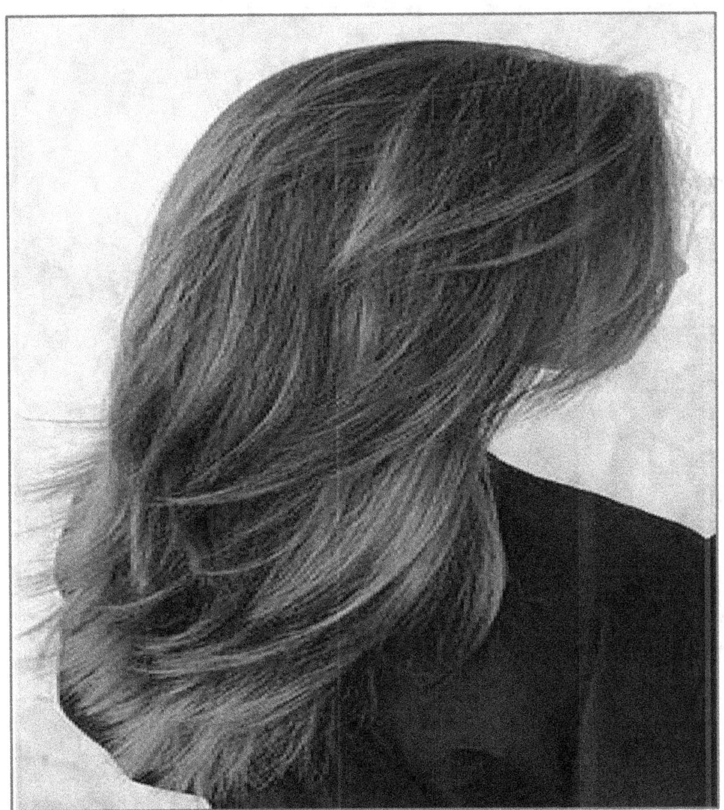

You want to be able to enhance the effect of the hair layers you cut. Modest highlights should be placed at the ends of your light layers. You'll see more depth and colour in your hair. You also get to show off your beautifully cut layers!

Brunette Long Layered Locks

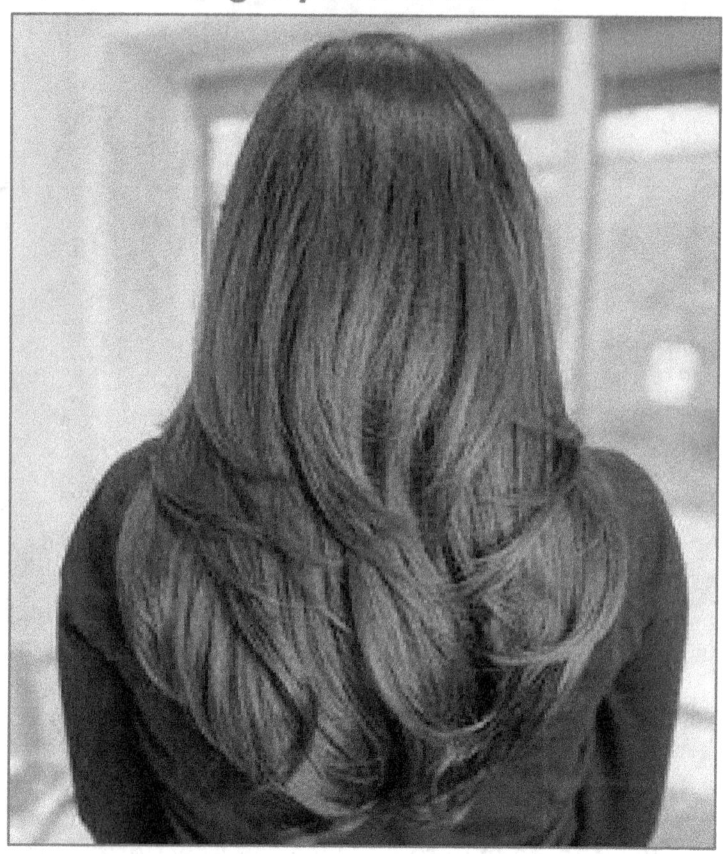

Who thinks brown hair looks boring? Long layers starting around mid-shaft may give your U-shaped cut movement and volume, making it sassier and more stylish. Feel free to experiment with different layer lengths for the best results.

Layers for Long Thick Hair

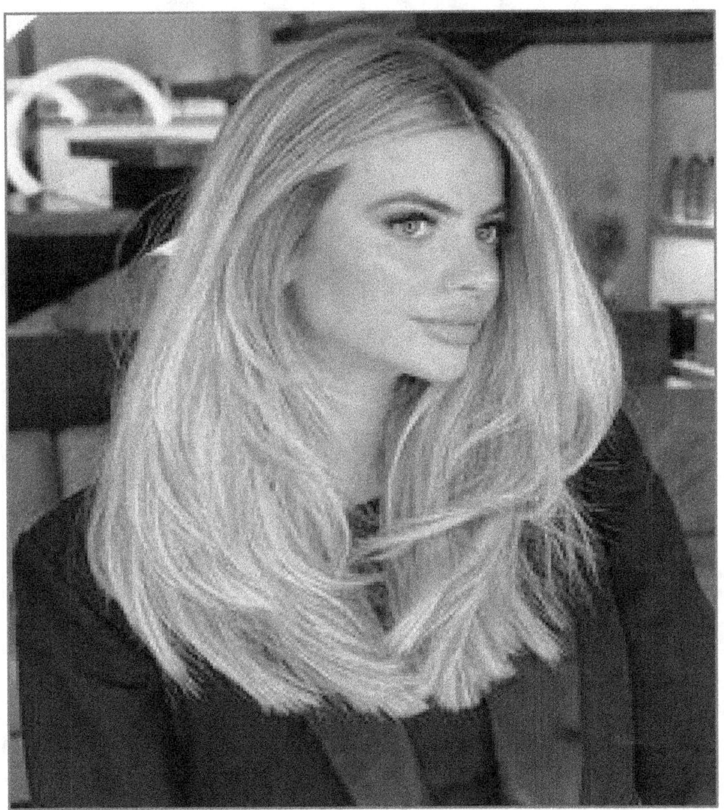

Your thick hair may be improved with a stylish centre part and a modern long layered haircut. Ask your hairdresser to create this wonderful golden balayage and flip the ends of your strands to add movement to make your hair seem light and dynamic.

Long Layered Brunette Hair with Curled Ends

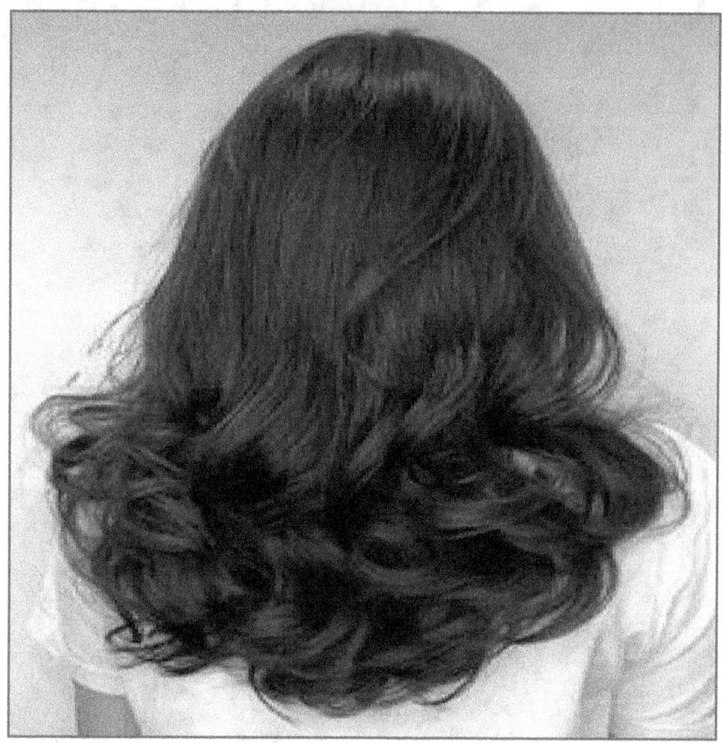

Long layered hair with bangs is a fashionable appearance that flatters textures ranging from straight to wavy. When the hair is cut short, curls have a tendency to bounce upward creating a "moppy" fringe. These cuts provide an extra touch of refinement and are easy to style into updos and downdos when the bangs are blow-dried or straightened.

Wrapping Feathered Layers Along the Sides

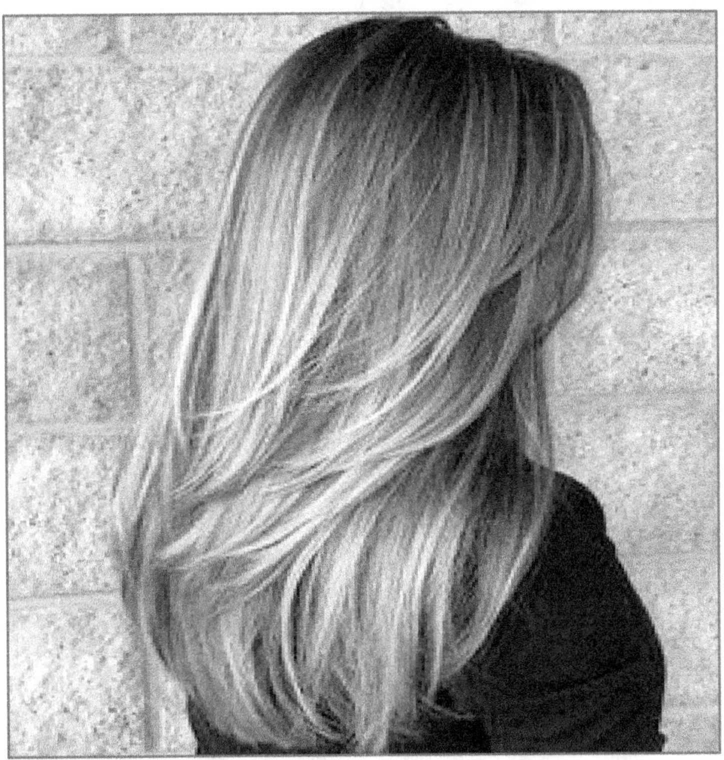

The most fashionable appearances are those that seem as if you merely rolled out of bed and went. You may get the ideal carefree image with long layers. By making it easy for your hair to fall into place, the feathery style saves you a ton of time in the morning.